Eat Smart, Lose Weight:
Understanding and Navigating Obesity

BY

Dr. Micheal E. Paschal

COPYRIGHT

TABLE OF CONTENT

INTRODUCTION

The modern-day obesity epidemic

Recently, it has become clear that over the past 20 years, obesity prevalence in the United States and other nations has been rising quickly. All age groups, both sexes and different ethnic groups, have been affected by this change. Due to the potential for detrimental effects on their morbidity and mortality as young adults, the rising prevalence in children and adolescents is especially concerning.

Obesity is unquestionably linked to a relative increase in conditions like osteoarthritis, diabetes, cardiovascular disease, several cancers, sleep disorders, gallbladder disease, and diabetes. It also negatively affects many other conditions, including urinary stress incontinence, menstrual disorders, psychological disorders, and pregnancy complications. It is a crucial part of the metabolic syndrome, which is emerging as a significant cluster of risk factors for cardiovascular disease.

It will be necessary to mobilize various stakeholders and allocate sufficient resources to combat this epidemic. These strategies need to be implemented immediately.

Thousands of articles about the rise in obesity prevalence in recent years have been published in popular magazines, scientific journals, and newspapers. In terms of the severity of its detrimental effects on public health, the issue has been referred to as an epidemic and contrasted with the perils of alcohol and tobacco use. Furthermore, the importance of children and adolescents in this change has become apparent as the full extent of the population's relatively quick increase in weight has been recognized. It's intriguing to think about why the rise in obesity in the population over the past two decades has suddenly come to be seen as something that could be so dangerous. Whatever the case, there is no denying the gravity of the obesity epidemic and the urgent need to develop strategies to treat those who have the disorder and lower the prevalence of obesity in the population in the future.

The Difficulties of Losing Weight in a High-Calorie Environment

They face numerous obstacles that make losing weight difficult for them.

The most significant difficulties people encounter when attempting to lose weight are:

- maintaining one's resolve
- a lack of motivation.
- eating healthy foods
- and overcoming hunger

Part I:

Understanding the Science of Obesity

CHAPTER 1

What do overweight and obesity mean?

Obsessive and overweight behaviors are characterized by abnormal or excessive fat accumulation that may have adverse health effects.

Body mass index (BMI) is a straightforward weight-for-height metric frequently used to categorize adults who are overweight or obese. It is calculated by dividing an individual's weight in kilograms by the square of their height in meters (kg/m2).

The World Health Organization defines obesity and overweight in adults as follows.

Overweight is defined as having a BMI of 25 or higher.

• A body mass index (BMI) of 30 is considered obese.

Because BMI is consistent across all adult ages and all sexes, it offers the most useful population-level measure of overweight and obesity. It should be regarded as a rough guide, though, as different people may have different degrees of fatness.

When classifying children as overweight or obese, age must be considered.

For kids younger than five years old:

Weight-for-height greater than two standard deviations above the Child Growth Standards median is considered overweight.
• If a person's weight is more than three standard deviations above the Child Growth Standards median, they are considered obese.

The following definitions apply to children between the ages of 5 and 19: overweight and obesity.

A BMI for an age greater than one standard deviation above the Growth Reference median is considered overweight.
• The obesity rate is over two standard deviations above the Growth Reference median.

Overweight and obesity: what causes them?

Being overweight and obese are primarily caused by an energy imbalance between calories expended and consumed. It is well known that imbalances between the energy obtained from food and the energy used to sustain life and carry out physical labor cause changes in body weight. There have been the following worldwide.

• consuming more foods heavy in fat and sugar that are high in energy; and.
• a rise in inactivity brought on by shifting transportation options, growing urbanization, and the passive nature of many occupations.

Alterations in dietary and physical activity habits are frequently brought about by changes in the environment and society brought about by development, as well as by the absence of policies that promote these changes in areas like health, agriculture, transportation, urban planning, environment, food processing, distribution, marketing, and education.

What are the usual health effects of obesity and overweight?

A raised BMI is one of the main risk factors for non-communicable diseases.

In 2012, cardiovascular diseases were the primary cause of death, primarily heart disease and stroke.
• diabetes.
• musculoskeletal conditions, particularly osteoarthritis, a degenerative disease of the joints that is highly incapacitating.
• a few cancers, such as those of the endometrium, breast, ovary, prostate, liver, gallbladder, kidney, and colon.

As BMI rises, so does the risk for these non-communicable diseases.

There is a correlation between childhood obesity and an increased risk of obesity, early mortality, and disability in adulthood. However, obese children also have higher risks for breathing problems, fractures, hypertension, early indicators of cardiovascular disease, insulin resistance, psychological effects, and early markers of cardiovascular disease.

What is the best way to decrease obesity and overweight? Obesity and overweight are primarily avoidable, as are the non-communicable diseases associated with them. To prevent overweight and obesity, supportive environments and communities play a crucial role in influencing people's decisions by making the selection of healthier foods and regular physical activity the most straightforward option (i.e., the most readily available, affordable, and easy to make).

Individuals can:

• Reduce the amount of energy obtained from total sugars and fats.

• eat more fruits, vegetables, nuts, whole grains, and legumes.

• Take regular physical exercise; adults should aim for 150 minutes per week, while children should get 60 minutes daily.

People's ability to live a healthy lifestyle is a prerequisite for the full impact of individual responsibility. For this reason, society must encourage people to heed the advice above by persistently enacting population- and evidence-based policies that make regular physical activity and healthier eating options quickly and affordably available to all, especially the most vulnerable. A tax on beverages with added sugar is one instance of such a policy.

The following are some crucial ways that the food industry can support the promotion of healthy diets:

• lowering processed foods' fat, sugar, and salt contents.
• guaranteeing that all customers have access to and can afford various healthful and nourishing options.
• restricting marketing of foods heavy in fats, sugars, and salt, particularly those sold to kids and teenagers.
• Make sure that various healthful food options are available and encourage frequent physical activity at work.

CHAPTER 2

The relationship between the mind and body

Our biological functioning can be influenced either positively or negatively by our thoughts, feelings, beliefs, and attitudes. Put another way, our bodies' levels of health can be affected by our thoughts.

Conversely, our mental state can be influenced (positively or negatively) by our physical actions, including our diet, level of exercise, and posture. As a result, our bodies and minds have intricate relationships.

The concept of the mind-body link has been introduced previously. Until about 300 years ago, the mind and body were treated as one in almost every medical system worldwide. However, the idea that the mind and body are two separate entities began to take hold in the West during the 17th century. According to this perspective, the body had no relationship to the mind and was more like a machine with interchangeable, independent parts.

There were unquestionable advantages to this Western perspective, which laid the groundwork for advancements in allopathic medicine, including surgery, trauma care, and pharmaceuticals. It also minimized humans' innate capacity for healing and drastically curtailed scientific research into their emotional and spiritual lives.

Gradually, this perspective began to shift in the 20th century. Scholars commenced investigating the correlation between the mind and body, presenting intricate connections through scientific demonstrations.

Emotional Consumption and Food Needs.

You're not the only one who runs to the pantry when you feel low or unhappy. When faced with intense, challenging emotions, people often seek solace in food.

It is known as emotional eating, when you eat to deal with your feelings. At times, everyone engages in it.

For our bodies to survive, we must eat. It makes sense that eating activates the brain's reward system and improves mood.

Emotional eating may become problematic if it occurs frequently and you have no other coping mechanisms.

Food doesn't solve the real problem, even though it might seem like a way to cope with those situations. Food won't make you feel better if you're depressed, lonely, tense, bored, or exhausted.

It can be difficult for some people to deal with the guilt and shame that come with this cycle of using food as a coping mechanism.

So much of what we do revolves around food. A component of our festivities is food. A thoughtful gesture of caring is preparing food for someone who is struggling. You can build connections by sharing food with other people.

Feelings associated with food are normal.

The aim is to enable you to choose what, when, and how you eat consciously. There will be occasions when using food as a coping mechanism makes sense. There are more effective coping mechanisms for other situations.

What triggers an individual's emotional eating behavior?

The need to eat can be sparked by almost anything. Typical outside causes of emotional eating could be:

Workplace stress.

• Concerns about money.

• Medical conditions.

• Problems with relationships.

Emotional eating is more common in those who have followed restrictive diets or have a history of dieting.

Other possible internal reasons are:

• Not being able to reflect on oneself (realizing how you feel).

• alexithymia is the inability to recognize, comprehend, or articulate feelings.

• dysregulation of emotions (inability to control emotions).

• underactive cortisol response to stress due to a reversed hypothalamic pituitary adrenal (HPA) stress axis.

Emotional eating is frequently a habitual behavior. The habit gets more ingrained as food is used as a coping mechanism.

Does emotional eating qualify as a disorder of eating?

An eating disorder cannot be diagnosed based solely on emotional eating. That might be an indication of disordered eating, which has the potential to turn into an eating disorder.

The following are examples of disordered eating.

• imposing strict dietary guidelines.

• classifying food as "good" or "bad".

• Restrictions on food or frequent dieting.

• frequently eating to satisfy feelings rather than actual hunger.

• irregular times for meals.

• Food-related obsessions that become so strong that they start to affect your entire life.

• Guilt or shame after consuming what you consider to be "unhealthy" foods.

According to the Academy of Nutrition and Dietetics, the diagnosis of eating disorders is made when a person's eating habits match specific criteria. Many people who don't fit the criteria for an eating disorder nevertheless engage in disordered eating behaviors.

To get help, you don't need an eating disorder diagnosis. You ought to enjoy a positive relationship with food.

How come food?

Eating turns into a coping mechanism for a variety of reasons. An emotional void or a sense of emptiness can result from difficult emotions.

Dopamine is a neurotransmitter that is released into the brain when we eat.

With food, we also form routines and habits. If you eat whenever you're stressed, you might not even realize that you're reaching for food when stress arises.

Moreover, food is widely available and lawful. You may become more hungry if you see or hear messages about food.

Comparing emotional vs. physical yearning.

To survive, humans require food. Needing food and wanting particular flavors or textures is a natural human behavior.

How to distinguish between physical and emotional hunger cues may need to be clarified. It may be challenging. There are occasions when both are combined.

Emotional eating is more common if you haven't eaten in several hours or need to eat more throughout the day.

You can distinguish between the two by using these hints.

What symptoms indicate emotional eating?

Individuals who eat emotionally might feel the following;

• unhinged when it comes to particular meals.

• a strong emotional craving for food.

A constant desire to consume food despite not being physically hungry.

• as if eating soothes or pleases them.

Methods for quitting emotional eating.

Emotional eating is a habit that is difficult to break, but it is doable. Here are a few coping mechanisms for you.

Open a journal of feelings.

It's better if you are more aware of your habits. Food can naturally be consumed in reaction to feelings—your chances of making changes increase with your understanding of how you feel about specific actions.

When you eat but are not truly hungry, try keeping a journal of those instances. Keep in mind:

• the circumstances.

• Your state of mind.

• Any feelings that surfaced during the urge to eat.

Consider including a space for you to write down what you accomplished. Did you eat as soon as possible, wait a while, or find another way to pass the time?

Aim to avoid passing judgment on your results. When you eat to satisfy your emotions, be genuinely curious about what's happening.

It requires a lot of practice to do this. As you begin your exploration, treat yourself with kindness. Perfectionism is not needed.

Look for alternate coping mechanisms.

You can begin to make changes once you know more about the feelings, circumstances, or ideas that can set off an eating episode.

If you've noticed that you always eat when stressed, you should address the stress. Consider a few strategies you can use to reduce your stress.

If you find that you snack when you're bored, think about strategies for handling your idle time. What other activities could you engage in to pass the time?

Retraining your mind to focus on other activities instead of reaching for food requires patience and repetition. Try a variety of approaches to see what suits you the best.

Exert your body.

One effective strategy for reducing stress and anxiety is to move your body.

Stress hormone levels in your body can be lowered with exercise. Additionally, it releases endorphins, which improve your mood. Training can assist in addressing the underlying emotional factors that lead to overeating.

It's not required to be very intense. If you're not exercising right now, think about going for a five-minute walk or doing light stretching. Take note of your feelings towards this.

Movements that promote mindfulness, such as yoga, have an additional advantage. Regular yoga practitioners report generally reduced levels of stress and anxiety.

Mindful consumption of food.

It is an eating style where choices about what to eat are made based on internal cues. Eating mindfully has been linked to psychological well-being and effectively improves your relationship with food.

You can savor the act of eating to the fullest. It invites you to take your time and pay closer attention to the food's flavors, textures, aromas, and sounds.

Preparing food in advance and thoroughly examining what is needed at that precise moment is the essence of mindful eating. Is it food? If yes, what kind of food? If not, what else will satisfy this need?

Being an attentive eater requires time and patience.

The following is taken into account when eating mindfully:

• Examines the meal's broader context, including the food source, the method of preparation, and the person who handled it.

• recognizes cues from both inside and outside the body that influence our appetite.

As we eat, we take note of the food's appearance, flavor, aroma, and physical sensation.

• Recognizes the physical sensations following a meal.

• conveys thanks for the meal.

• Before or following the meal, try deep breathing exercises or mindfulness.

• considers our foods' impact on the environment locally and globally.

Seven mindful dining techniques;

1. Respect the cuisine.

Recall who cooked the meal and where the food was grown. To enhance the dining experience, try to avoid distractions while eating.

2. Make use of all your senses.

As you eat, pay attention to the flavors, textures, aromas, colors, and sounds of the food and your feelings. To use these senses, take occasional breaks.

3. Portion out the food carefully.

By doing this, food waste and overeating may be prevented. Only fill a dinner plate that is no bigger than nine inches across.

4. Chew everything thoroughly and savor tiny portions.

By doing so, you'll be able to savor the meal's flavors more slowly and thoroughly.

5. To prevent overindulging, eat slowly.

Eating slowly increases your chances of identifying when you are about 80% full or feeling satisfied, at which point you can stop eating.

6. Eat every day.

Extended fasting heightens the likelihood of intense hunger, which could prompt a hasty and less nutritious meal choice. Reducing these risks involves scheduling meals for roughly the same time each day and allowing enough time to enjoy a meal or snack.

7. Consume a plant-based diet for the environment and your health.

Think about how certain foods will affect you down the road. Saturated fat and processed meat have been linked to an increased risk of heart disease and colon cancer. Environmental damage is caused during the production of animal-based foods like dairy and meat than plant-based foods.

CHAPTER 3

Hormones and Metabolism.

Endocrine glands produce trace amounts of hormones, which are non-nutrient chemicals that function as intercellular messengers. Hormones are then released into the bloodstream and carried to a distant target organ. Hormones are in charge of controlling metabolism in addition to offering chemical coordination, integration, and regulation in the human body. Some hormones can slow your metabolism, while others can speed it up.
The metabolism process is how living things obtain and use the free energy needed to perform their essential life functions. It might directly or indirectly impact how you feel throughout the day, how much weight you gain, and how energetic you are. Many variables, such as age, sex, muscle mass, and physical activity, affect metabolism or BMR (Basal Metabolic Rate), with some people having a fast metabolism and others having a slow one.

What Are Hormones, and How Do They Affect Metabolism?

Endocrine glands are specialized glands that synthesize and produce hormones, which are like messengers for our body and are used to control and regulate the activity of particular cells and organs. The thyroid, adrenal, pancreas, parathyroid, thymus, and gonads (testis and ovary) are among the endocrine glands that produce hormones, along with the hypothalamus, pituitary, and pineal. Aside from these, a few other organs, e.g., the kidney, heart, and gastrointestinal tract. , which also create hormones.

Health and proper bodily functions, including metabolism, are produced by a healthy hormonal balance. Contrarily, hormonal imbalance can cause metabolism to slow down, which can lead to weight gain. Numerous hormones, including cortisol, thyroid hormones, and testosterone, directly impact metabolism.

Different Hormones and Their Function in Metabolism.
Our bodies depend on hormones, which control almost everything, including growth, mood, behavior, digestion, and fertility. Your hormones are in charge of making sure you stay healthy and function properly. The endocrine glands produce various hormones that control metabolism in multiple ways. The essential hormones that regulate metabolism are:
1. Insulin.
2. Testosterone.
3. hormones that affect the thyroid.
4. ghrelin and leptin.
5. the hormone cortisol.

How the metabolism affects weight loss.
The internal process by which your body expends energy and burns calories is known as metabolism. It works round-the-clock to keep your body active, even when you're resting or sleeping,

by converting the food and nutrients you eat into the energy your body needs to breathe, circulate blood, grow and repair cells, and perform all the other tasks necessary for survival. Different people experience this process with varying degrees of intensity. Your genes largely determine how quickly your metabolism functions.

People can have a fast, slow, or average metabolism regardless of body size and composition.

Age also impacts metabolism because, even if you start out with a fast metabolism, it can slow down with time. The ease or difficulty with which people gain or lose weight reflects differences in metabolism speed. Some people struggle to lose weight by cutting calories because they have a slow metabolism, which burns fewer calories and causes more to be stored as fat. People with fast metabolisms burn calories more quickly, which explains why some people can eat a lot without gaining weight.

Can a slow metabolism be made to work more quickly?
Your metabolism is something you can control. A minor adjustment is frequently all it takes to increase your calorie burn. That could give people the extra push they require to lose and maintain weight, make a change to a healthier diet, and ensure they get enough exercise. As an illustration:

Speed things up.
Increase your regular exercise routine with some high-intensity interval training. Your metabolism can remain stimulated after

an interval training session for a full day. For instance, if you're walking or jogging outside or on a treadmill, speed up for 30 to 60 seconds, then slow down to your regular pace. Repeat this cycle eight to twelve times.

Consume protein and lift weights.
The thermic effect of food is the term used to describe how your metabolism increases whenever you consume, digest, and store food. Protein has a higher thermic effect because protein takes longer to digest and absorb by your body than fats and carbohydrates.

Sup green tea.
According to studies, Epigallocatechin gallate, a substance found in green tea, has been linked to increased fat and calorie burning.

The role of hormones in obesity.
Chemical messengers known as hormones control bodily functions. They contribute to the problem of obesity. The hormones leptin and insulin, sex hormones, and growth hormones impact our appetite, metabolism (the rate at which our body burns calories for energy), and how much body fat we have in different parts of our bodies. These hormones are present in higher amounts in obese people, which promotes an abnormal metabolism and the buildup of body fat.

The endocrine system, a network of glands, secretes hormones into our bloodstream. To help our body handle various situations and stresses, the endocrine system collaborates with the nervous and immune systems. Obesity can result from hormonal excesses or deficiencies, and vice versa; obesity can result from hormonal changes.

Leptin and obesity.
Fat cells produce the hormone leptin, which is then released into the bloodstream. Leptin decreases a person's appetite by influencing particular brain regions that control the desire to eat. Additionally, it has a say in how the body handles its fat reserves.
Leptin is produced by fat, so individuals with obesity typically have higher leptin levels than those with average weight.
Despite having higher levels of this hormone that curbs appetite, obese people are less sensitive to its effects and, as a result, tend not to experience satiety during and after meals. The reason why leptin messages are not reaching obese people's brains is still being investigated.

Insulin and obesity.
The pancreas secretes the hormone insulin, which is crucial for controlling the metabolism of fat and carbohydrates. In tissues like muscles, the liver, and fat, insulin stimulates the uptake of glucose (sugar) from the blood. This process is crucial to ensure

that there is energy available for daily activity and to keep blood glucose levels within normal range.

Sometimes, in an obese person, the ability of tissues to control glucose levels is lost due to a loss of insulin signals. Type II diabetes and the metabolic syndrome may develop due to this.

Sexual hormones and obesity.

The distribution of body fat is crucial in the emergence of obesity-related illnesses like heart disease, stroke, and some types of arthritis. Compared to fat stored on our hips, thighs, and bottom, abdominal fat is a more significant risk factor for disease. Estrogens and androgens play a role in determining how body fat is distributed. The ovaries in premenopausal women produce the sex hormones known as estrogens. Every cycle of a woman's menstrual cycle triggers ovulation.

In their testes (testicles) or ovaries, men and postmenopausal women do not produce a lot of estrogen. Instead, a large portion of their estrogen is produced in their body fat, albeit in much smaller amounts than in their premenopausal ovaries. Androgen production in the testes is high in younger men. These levels gradually decrease with age in men.

The distribution of body fat changes along with aging, and this is true for both men and women's sex hormone levels. Older men and postmenopausal women tend to increase fat storage around their abdomen (making them "apple-shaped"). In contrast, women of childbearing age tend to store fat in their lower body (making them "pear-shaped"). Women who are taking estrogen supplements after menopause do not develop belly fat. Animal studies have also demonstrated the excessive weight gain caused by a lack of estrogen.

Glucocorticoids and obesity.

Growth hormone, which affects a person's height and promotes the development of bone and muscle, is produced by the pituitary gland in our brain. Growth hormone has an impact on metabolism, or how quickly we use up energy-containing calories. According to research, obese individuals have lower growth hormone levels than healthy-weight individuals.

Obesity and inflammatory components.

Low-grade chronic inflammation within the fat tissue is another aspect of obesity. Adipose (fat) tissue immune cells and pro-inflammatory factors are released from fat cells themselves due to stress reactions that occur within fat cells due to excessive fat storage.

Obesity hormones as a disease risk factor.

Obesity is linked to a higher risk of developing several illnesses, such as cardiovascular disease, stroke, and cancer. It is also linked to decreased longevity (a shorter life expectancy) and a lower quality of life. For instance, increased estrogen production in the fat of older obese women is linked to a higher risk of breast cancer, proving the significance of the source of estrogen production.

Behavior and hormones linked to obesity.

Hormone concentrations in obese people promote the buildup of body fat. The processes that control appetite and body fat distribution appear to be "reset" over time by behaviors like binge eating and infrequent exercise, increasing a person's physiological propensity to gain weight. The body fights against temporary disruptions like crash dieting because it constantly attempts to maintain balance.

There is a decrease in blood leptin after a low-calorie diet, according to numerous studies. A person's appetite may increase, and their metabolism may slow down if their leptin levels are low. This may help to explain why people who follow crash diets frequently put on the weight they lost. Although more research is required before this becomes a reality, leptin therapy may one day assist dieters in long-term weight maintenance.

There is proof that consistent behavior changes, like eating well and working out regularly, can re-train the body to burn excess body fat and keep it off. Studies have also demonstrated that losing weight through a healthy diet, regular exercise, or bariatric surgery improves insulin sensitivity, reduces inflammation, and advantageous obesity hormone modulation. Additionally, losing weight is linked to a lower risk of heart disease, stroke, type II diabetes, and some types of cancer.

CHAPTER 4

Weight gain and genetics

A person may gain weight more quickly than others in some cases due to bad genes rather than poor diet.

Scientists have discovered that gene variants that cause people to feel less full after eating may be more widespread than previously believed, causing those who carry these gene variants to eat more frequently or consume more calorie-dense foods.

It is not in your control to be overweight. By definition, the genetics of body weight also include the genetics of how our brains regulate our food intake.

The National Health and Nutrition Examination Survey estimates that nearly a third of American adults and almost one in every six kids and teenagers between the ages of two and 19 are overweight. Among the two in five obese adults in America, type 2 diabetes, high blood pressure, stroke, cardiovascular disease, and some forms of cancer are just a few of the conditions at increased risk due to this excess weight. If our weight is determined by our genes rather than our lifestyle, what is the root of this epidemic?

While the type of food consumed and the level of physical activity play a significant role in the rising number of obese people, science is now showing that similar to height, between

50 and 80 percent of the variation in body weight can be attributed to subtle changes in some genes. The hundreds of genetic variations that each have a tiny impact and make some of us slightly more susceptible to gaining weight are more common than the rare single genetic mutations that make obesity inevitable. When a person inherits several of these variations, their risk of obesity rises noticeably, especially when other lifestyle factors are considered.

Parental obesity is the leading risk factor for childhood and adolescent obesity. If both parents are obese, the risk is incredibly high. The inheritance of obesity, however, rarely adheres to the standard Mendelian patterns. Various gene mutations, deletions, and single nucleotide polymorphisms influence obesity. Most cases are polygenic, a result of multiple genes interacting with a changing environment. Although individual "obesity genes" only have a minor impact on phenotype, inherited genetic variations significantly affect body mass and how the body maintains a healthy balance between nutrition and exercise. While polygenic inheritance is most frequently linked to obesity, there are other situations where the cause is monogenic or syndromic. In most cases, monogenic obesity is caused by a single gene mutation, with severe obesity as the primary symptom. On the other hand, symptomatic obesity has a variety of traits, and obesity is one of them.

"monogenic obesity" refers to obesity caused by a single gene mutation. In these situations, a single gene variant is sufficient to result in obesity in societies with plenty of food. Patients with monogenic obesity typically display extremely severe phenotypes that are characterized by the onset of obesity in childhood and are frequently accompanied by other behavioral, developmental, or endocrine disorders, such as hyperphagia and hypogonadism. However, severe developmental delays are uncommon.

Patients with syndromic obesity exhibit clinical obesity, mental retardation, dysmorphic features, and abnormal developmental patterns specific to particular organs. These disorders have a Mendelian genetic basis.

The most prevalent type of obesity—polygenic obesity—affects most obese children and results from a person's genetic predisposition to an environment that favors energy consumption over energy expenditure.

Genes that encode peptides intended to transmit hunger and satiety signals, genes involved in adipocyte growth and differentiation, and genes in charge of regulating energy expenditure are some of the genes connected to the etiology of obesity. 1.

Techniques for Solving Genetic Problems.

It is possible to partially combat a genetic predisposition to obesity by.

Diet modifications.

Fat and excess weight can build up when a person consumes more calories than they expend. This may result in weight gain in the long run.

Foods to eat and foods to avoid.

A person can lose weight by eating more whole grains and other high-fiber foods, such as fresh fruits and vegetables, and less processed, refined, and ready-made food high in sugar and fat. Whole grain and healthy fat-focused eating regimens, like the Mediterranean diet, are known to support healthy weight loss. In addition to lowering the risk of some metabolic syndrome-related diseases, fiber, and whole grains can also help. Type 2 diabetes, high blood pressure, and cardiovascular issues are all symptoms of the condition known as metabolic syndrome. The prevalence is higher in obese individuals.

Consistency.

Consistently adhering to a healthy diet is the most crucial component. Extremely low-calorie and restrictive diets may aid short-term weight loss, but long-term adherence is poor.

Severe restriction can result in nutritional deficiencies and unhelpful weight gain after the diet.
A doctor or dietitian can suggest a strategy and likely an effective weight-loss program.

Physical exercise.
Increasing activity levels along with dietary changes can assist people in achieving and maintaining a healthy weight while also enhancing mobility and mood.
There are many effective ways to begin being active.

- strolling quickly.
- Swimming.
- choosing to ascend rather than descend stairs.
- alighting a station earlier from a bus or train and continuing on foot.

To maintain weight, experts advise people to engage in two sessions of muscle-strengthening activity and at least 150 minutes of moderate-intensity exercise each week. Aim for 300 minutes or more of moderate-intensity exercise each week to lose weight.
A health professional should be consulted about how to begin exercising if a person is new to it or finds it challenging to be active because of health or mobility issues.
Medications for losing weight.
Medication such as: may be prescribed by a doctor.

- the Xenical drug orlistat.
- Qsymia, which contains the drugs phentermine and topiramate.
- Naltrexone and bupropion (Contrave).
- the medication liraglutide (Saxenda).
The drug semaglutide (Wegovy).
- the drug bremelanotide (IMCIVREE).

However, they typically only do this if weight loss has yet to be achieved through dietary changes and exercise or if the person's weight seriously threatens their health.
Medication should be used in conjunction with lifestyle changes, not instead of them.
GI symptoms, such as fatty stool and altered urination, are examples of side effects. The respiratory system, muscles, joints, headaches, and other organs have all been linked to unfavorable impacts by some.

Surgery.
To reduce food intake and calorie absorption, weight loss surgery may involve removing or altering a portion of the patient's stomach or small intestine.
This can assist a person in losing weight and lower their risk of developing high blood pressure, type 2 diabetes, and other metabolic syndrome symptoms accompanying obesity.
Surgery has the potential to bypass a portion of the digestive system or reduce the size of the stomach.

Gastric band or sleeve.
To reduce the size of the stomach, the surgeon uses a gastric sleeve or gastric band.

A gastric bypass.
In particular, the procedure can bypass the first portion of the small intestine's middle section. It also makes the stomach appear more petite.
This is typically more efficient than limiting procedures, but because the body can no longer absorb as many nutrients, there is a higher risk of vitamin and mineral deficiencies.

The use of hormones.
Small studies suggest hormone therapy may help obese and type 2 diabetic patients lose weight. New, non-surgical options might result from using these hormones.
However, more extensive studies are required to fully evaluate the effects of hormonal therapies for obesity because there is a shortage of research in the area.

Part II:
Navigating the High-Calorie World

CHAPTER 5.

Challenges with diet.

A healthy diet is crucial for maintaining weight control and preventing or treating many chronic conditions. However, maintaining a healthy diet necessitates meal planning and taking the time to shop and compare goods. Because of the above, some people may not eat as healthily as they should because eating healthier can occasionally mean spending more money at the grocery store. A registered dietitian can assist you in creating a plan that will fit your budget while lowering your risk of disease if you are having trouble eating healthfully.

Establishing New Habits.

Certain eating habits may have been formed during childhood, and eating is about more than just giving the body the calories and nutrients it needs. Food is sometimes used to deal with underlying emotions like boredom, anxiety, loneliness, etc. Eating is a social activity; some foods may be linked to good feelings. Begin by altering thought patterns like the need to finish everything on your plate and avoid wasting food, eating because you feel obligated to by friends or family, eating while multitasking, or eating because it makes you feel comfortable.

All the above factors can result in overeating and bad food decisions. Create alternative ways of thinking and coping, and gradually alter your habits by focusing on one trigger at a time.

Time is short.

Unhealthy food choices may result from a busy lifestyle and eating on the go. When you have the time, grabbing whatever is nearby can lead to poor eating habits. Go through your refrigerator and cabinets to remove unhealthy food and replace it with more wholesome alternatives. Plan and purchase already-cut meats and vegetables to save time preparing food. Select canned produce that hasn't added salt or sugar and has been preserved in juice or water. According to the Cleveland Clinic, heat, light, and air can all deplete the nutrients in fruit and vegetables. As a result, it is often preferable to purchase canned or frozen versions packed as soon as they are taken out of the ground. Make larger portions of your meals when you cook and freeze some to always have food on hand. You can avoid going to the store by ordering groceries online and delivering them to your house. You can save time and effort by doing these things, making it simpler to eat healthily.

Too much data.

There is a wealth of information about what eating healthily entails in the news, magazines, and online, making it difficult to distinguish what is real from what is false. So many diets promise to help you drop pounds quickly or manage conditions like heart disease and other illnesses. Americans consume too many calories and excessive amounts of bad fats, sugar, salt, and refined grains. Most people do not consume enough healthy fats, fiber, calcium, potassium, or vitamin D. Three to five servings of fruits and vegetables per day—each equal to one cup—are recommended for a well-balanced diet. Read nutrition labels and try to consume at least 1,500 mg of sodium daily and 25 to 35 g of fiber daily. A maximum of 30% of your daily calories should come from fat, with unsaturated fats making up most of that amount. The time and effort required to plan a menu can be challenging, but it is well worth it.

Cost.

Eating healthy can be difficult when you're on a tight budget because junk food is less expensive than healthy food. Learn to make a grocery list before you go to the store and to stock your pantry with necessities. To be ready and have a list to follow, look through the supermarket circulars, clip coupons, and find the sales. Since meat can be pricey, try going without meat for one or two meals a week. Instead, choose a dinner based on vegetables, beans, or whole grains. Find out if your grocery store offers a rewards card to accumulate points toward discounts. The tips mentioned above can result in significant financial savings and promote healthier eating.

Finding Hidden Calories.

Hidden calories are calories present in some foods, food products, and ingredients. However, they are not readily apparent to the consumer as calories or are purposefully disregarded as calories but still add to the daily caloric intake. The consumer is unaware of the calories, chooses to ignore them, or cannot see or recognize them, which is why they are referred to as "hidden" calories.

The traits of hidden calories are as follows:

• The majority people who eat food containing hidden calories are unaware of the foods' calorie counts.

• The names of the foods, their appearance, their taste, or general knowledge do not make them immediately apparent as high in calories or a high source of calories in the consumer's diet plan. For instance, some foods may be high in carbohydrates but have a bland flavor that hides their sugar content.

• When consuming the food or estimating the number of calories they will consume each day, consumers fail to consider the caloric content of such foods.

• Dieters often mistakenly think they are eating well or "eating healthy" when, in reality, they are consuming too many calories due to hidden calories.

• Because they are consumed continuously, or through mindless eating, hidden calories in food often add up quickly and cause

weight gain. g. Before the conclusion of a football game, such as the Super Bowl or the World Cup for soccer, several packets of corn chips, potato chips, and nachos can be consumed.
• Because the food is combined with well-known healthy foods and ingredients that are marketed in the media as "superfoods," "healthy," and "natural," the consumer minimizes the caloric effect of the food or overlooks its caloric content.
• A few customers mistakenly think a menu's healthy items will balance or enhance the unhealthy options. As a result, large quantities of unhealthy food with hidden calories are consumed.
• Sometimes, low-calorie foods with hidden calories are thought to be "too small to harm anyone" because they come in small packages. The result is that they are overly consumed.
• Most of the time, only a knowledgeable nutritionist, dietitian, or concerned consumer can identify foods with hidden calories.

Sources of hidden calories in food.
Many consume calories throughout the day that we may not even think to count or include in our daily calorie intake. Consider these sources for hidden calories in your diet to reach a 10-pound weight gain in a year with just 100 extra calories consumed daily:

• If you add cream and sugar to your coffee, you might be adding calories in addition to sweetness. Coffee is often necessary for many of us as a morning wake-me-up and occasionally an afternoon pick-me-up. You add about 15 calories for every teaspoon of sugar. Pay attention to the serving size when purchasing creamer. A serving of creamer typically contains two tablespoons, but if you pour it from a bottle, you're likely using much more. A simple way to cut these calories is by selecting non-fat milk and a sugar substitute. Dark-roasted coffees also have a bitter flavor profile and need cream and sweeteners to be drinkable. By utilizing lighter coffees and using less sugar and creamer per cup, you may be able to lower your calorie intake.

• Snacks with low protein content, such as yogurt, won't satisfy your hunger. Many food products that you might expect to give you energy might unless you eat a lot of them, which frequently defeats the purpose of getting enough energy to get through the day.

• We can sacrifice calories for flavor when using condiments. Pay attention to how much butter, mayonnaise, sour cream, ranch, and other ingredients there are. You apply. To find the serving size for each food, look at the nutrition facts label on the package. Always keep in mind that the calorie count is for one serving. You will consume twice as many calories if you use twice as much as a serving size.

Try replacing your higher-calorie favorites with these:

• Put hot sauce on your morning eggs rather than ketchup.

• Use plain Greek yogurt without added fat instead of sour cream when serving baked potatoes.
• For your vegetable dip, use salsa rather than ranch.
• Take non-bitter coffee with a light or medium roast into consideration.
• Substitutes for yogurt and dairy products high in energy (and protein per serving).
Reducing your intake of those sneaky calories and improving your health by making informed eating decisions can be accomplished by making minor changes to your diet over time.

Making Knowledgeable Food Decisions.

The consumption of food can be decided upon with knowledge. It's not a decision that's made in a vacuum. The person makes a wise decision based on knowledge that the consumer has acquired.

Information helps consumers understand their options when deciding whether to buy something or when selecting different foods. Data must be made available to improve the food market's transparency and allow consumers to judge, contrast, and choose foods following the essential values and preferences. Ten suggestions for selecting foods that will improve your health are provided below.

1. Instead of avoiding carbohydrates, choose healthy ones. Your best option is whole grains.
2. Examine the protein package carefully. The best options are fish, poultry, nuts, and beans.
3. Limit your intake of foods high in saturated fat and steer clear of foods containing trans fats. The best sources include nuts, fish, and plant oils.
4. Opt for a diet high in whole grains, vegetables, and fruits high in fiber.
5. Consume more fruits and vegetables. Choose dark green, yellow, orange, and red for color and variety.
6. Calcium is crucial. However, milk isn't the only or even the best source.
7. To quench your thirst, water is best. Avoid sugary beverages, and drink milk and juice in moderation.
8. Everyone's health is improved by consuming less salt. Fresh foods are better than processed ones, so choose more of them.
9. Drinking in moderation can be healthy, but not for everyone. It would help if you balanced the risks and benefits.
10. An excellent nutrition safety net is a daily multivitamin. An additional health boost could be provided by taking more vitamin D.

CHAPTER 6.

Convenience and fast food culture.

Fast food's definition.

Fast food is a well-liked option for many people searching for a quick and simple supper, whether on the road, working long hours, or just searching for a quick and affordable lunch. Franchises and chain restaurants have popped up all over the place due to the fast food industry's explosive growth over the past few decades. Fast food is frequently seen as a practical substitute for people who are too busy or need more resources to prepare meals at home.

Over 25 percent of American adults regularly eat fast food. However, a common trade-off for this convenience is fast food's lack of nutritional value. Fast food is frequently high in calories, fat, sugar, and salt and can contribute to some medical conditions, such as type 2 diabetes, obesity, and heart disease. In addition, many fast food establishments have come under fire for using ingredients that weren't sourced ethically, creating waste, and abusing resources that aggravated the environment. Despite these criticisms, many people still choose fast food, which impacts culture and society.

Various factors cause the United States' obsession with fast food. Fast food is so simple that you frequently don't even have to leave the comfort of your car to eat. The price of fast food is also extremely low; a Big Mac meal from McDonald's, which includes a burger, fries, and beverage, costs only $5.99. Lastly, obtaining a meal from a fast food restaurant is quick; in most cases, your food will be prepared and served in under 10 minutes. These are the leading causes of fast food's popularity in the US; as a result, it has been growing steadily for years and is expected to continue.

Convenience is a critical factor in the appeal of fast food. You can get an entire meal at a fast food restaurant in minutes rather than spending time preparing a meal in your kitchen and at the grocery store. The most well-known fast food chain, McDonald's, has over 37,000 locations, far outnumbering all others. One crucial aspect of McDonald's food's convenience is how it is served. The majority of McDonald's meals can be consumed with just your hands and don't require any type of cutlery. This implies that they can eat whenever and wherever they want. As a result, more than 20% of American meals are consumed in automobiles, a practice that was rare before the advent of fast food.

Methods for Finding Healthy Fast Food.

Frequenting fast food restaurants makes it very challenging to maintain a healthy diet. A single meal of fast food frequently contains enough calories, sodium, and unhealthy fat to last an entire day. Additionally, it often lacks fiber, fruit, and vegetables and is generally low in nutrients.

You are not required to avoid fast food in light of this altogether. Fast food can be a real lifesaver when you're rushing around and hungry. The best part is that it is convenient, affordable, and tasty. While occasionally giving in to a craving is acceptable, it cannot become a habit if you want to maintain your health.

Moderation is essential regarding how frequently you visit fast-food restaurants and what you order when you do.

When keeping an eye on your weight or your health, fast food menus can be challenging. Finding a nutritious, well-balanced meal in most fast-food establishments can be difficult. However, you can always make better decisions for your health than others. You can stay on track using the following advice and menu suggestions.

Your meal should contain no more than 500 calories overall.
The average adult consumes 836 calories in a fast food meal, which is 175 calories more than they think they do. Most chains provide nutritional information on their websites and at the franchise location, so avoid speculating. Use the knowledge provided.

Choosing foods with less fat, protein, and fiber is a good idea. Try to find foods that contain healthier ingredients, such as whole grains, fiber, and high-quality protein. Additionally, look for choices that are relatively low in saturated fats. Also, avoid anything with trans fats in it.

If you want a health boost, bring your supplements.

Even with careful ordering, it can be tricky to consume enough fiber and other necessary vitamins and nutrients from a fast food menu. If you prepare beforehand, you can bring wholesome sides and toppings like cottage cheese or yogurt, apple or pear slices, carrot sticks, dried fruit, nuts, and seeds.

Monitor your intake of sodium.

Cardiovascular disease is significantly influenced by high sodium intake. Adults should consume no more than 2,300 mg of sodium daily and no more than 1,500 mg, according to the American Heart Association. Unfortunately, even when eating lower-calorie meals while fasting, achieving that can still be challenging. Your best bet is to eat low-sodium meals before and after your fast food meal and prepare beforehand. You can lessen some of the harm by requesting that your burger or meat be prepared without additional salt.

You can make better decisions with the aid of guides.

On their websites, numerous fast-food chains provide nutritional information. These lists can be challenging to understand and use, but they are the best resource for current, accurate information on your menu options. Many other websites and apps also offer nutritional information, frequently in more user-friendly formats.

Consider lean meats that have been grilled or roasted.

Avoid fried or breaded foods, such as crispy chicken sandwiches and breaded fish fillets. Alternatively, go with lean roast beef, turkey, chicken breast, ham, or boneless ham. It would be best if you generally stuck to grilling skinless chicken.

Study the menu's descriptions carefully.
Usually, foods with the descriptions "deep-fried," "pan-fried," "basted," "breaded," "creamy," "crispy," "scaled," or "au gratin" have high sodium and unhealthy fat content. This also applies to sauces like Alfredo or cream.

Planning Your Meals in a Busy World.
Finding the time and energy to prepare healthy meals daily may be challenging in our busy lives. By planning and preparing, you can control your diet and ensure you're giving your body delicious and nourishing meals. You can have delicious and nutritious meals all week without going over budget with the right meal prep ideas. Meal preparation also improves your week by allowing you to try new flavors, save time, and make wiser decisions. These meal prep ideas will undoubtedly ease your life and improve your diet, whether you're a busy professional, student, or traveling parent.
Plan your meals according to these suggestions to maximize weight loss.

1. Make a menu plan.

To begin, make a plan for your meals for the upcoming week. Consider your dietary preferences, nutritional needs, and any goals you may have, such as weight loss or muscle growth. Prepare a menu that includes a range of proteins, whole grains, healthy fats, and colorful fruits and vegetables. Making plans will not only help you save time but will also help you make more informed decisions about your grocery purchases.

2. Get the ingredients ready in advance.

Spend some time in advance preparing the ingredients to make cooking during the week a breeze. Proteins should be marinated, while vegetables should be washed and chopped. Store each meal separately in a zip-top bag or container to make it simple to prepare them later. By not having to prepare things every day, you'll save time and be more motivated to stick to your healthy eating plan.

3. Add and subtract.

Create a range of components that can be mixed and matched all week. For example, prepare a large quantity of roasted vegetables, various proteins (chicken, tofu, or fish), and several sauces or dressings to add flavor. You can create new meals daily that satisfy your palate by combining these ingredients in various ways.

4. controlling portions.

Use portioned containers or meal prep containers with dividers to ensure portion control. You can avoid overeating and ensure that your meals are balanced by doing this. Divide your vegetables, cereals, and proteins into the appropriate serving sizes, leaving room for wholesome fats and sauces. If you prepare your meals in advance, you will have a clear reminder to guide your eating patterns and support your goals.

5. salads made in mason jars.

Using mason jars makes it easy and appealing to enjoy crisp, fresh salads all week long. On top of the dressing at the jar's bottom, layers of filling ingredients like grains, proteins, and vegetables should be added. Save the delicate greens for the top layer to avoid wilting. Shake the container to distribute the dressing before serving your salad.

6. Suitable for freezing meals.

Make freezer-friendly dishes that can be quickly reheated to maximize your freezer. Make enormous quantities of soups, stews, or casseroles and divide them for freezing. These meals could be beneficial on busy days when you don't have time to cook. Simply defrosting and heating them will enable you to prepare a healthy and mouthwatering supper quickly.

7. judicious snacking.

Remember to include snacks in your meal plans. Prepare time-saving, healthy snacks like homemade energy balls, pre-portioned nuts, and cut fruit. By keeping these snacks on hand, you can make better choices when hungry and avoid reaching for unhealthy options.

In conclusion, meal planning is crucial to overcoming the challenges of a busy lifestyle and ensuring you feed your body nourishing foods. Planning your meals, getting the ingredients ready in advance, and embracing techniques like mix-and-match, portion control, mason jar salads, freezer-friendly dishes, and smart snacking can help you save time, enjoy a variety of flavors, and make wise decisions for your health. By being organized and working hard, you can change your eating habits, maintain a healthy diet, and achieve your fitness goals. To enjoy the benefits of fast, healthy eating, make meal preparation a regular part of your life.

CHAPTER 7

Social and Environmental Factors

Effects of social eating

People eat differently when they eat alone and when they eat with others. In particular, we adhere to strict dietary standards like our fellow diners and eat in imitation of the foods and amounts consumed by our dining partners. Eating together and following similar cultural norms or rules is a source of unity and cultural identity that brings us closer together. There is much evidence that people like to eat with others and that social eating is more enjoyable and makes people happier. Not only does good food taste better when you eat it together, but eating it with people who like food and eat relatively large amounts of it also allows you to eat more without feeling like you've eaten in excess. In addition, people who share food seem to be friendlier to each other, and those who eat similar foods seem to feel more confident. However, some people find that eating alone is more comfortable, less stressful and gives them more autonomy over time. But despite these differences, all cultures value social eating, maybe because of the connectivity and positive impact.

Have you ever seen someone yawn?
Something similar happens when we eat with other people. We see them biting, and we do the same. This is called a behavioural

model. Behavioural modelling is when someone imitates the behaviour of another person. We can do this intentionally or even unintentionally. We can't altogether avoid the influence of others, but if we become more aware of these tendencies, we can take steps to guide our choices in better ways. How other people influence our food choices

We are often influenced by the food and drink choices of those around us. Research shows that when we eat with others, we tend to bite or swallow right after them. One study even found that moviegoers took a sip immediately after a movie character drank alcohol. This means that if the people around us eat and drink more, we may eat and drink more than we think. Some research suggests that you can choose your foods and how much you eat based on what you consider "normal" in a given situation. The perception that a food is normal has a more significant impact on choices than the perception that a food is healthy. For example, one study found that people who were told that eating vegetables was normal ate more vegetables than those told that vegetables were healthy.

We also tend to choose portion sizes based on our beliefs about what normal food looks like. For example, one study found that people would eat more cookies if others in the same research ate more.

The environment also plays a vital role in our food choices. We are more likely to copy our partner's eating habits in environments where we are not sure how much "normal" food we should be eating.

For example, we are likelier to imitate what our peers eat in unstructured settings, such as snacking at happy hour or watching a movie, than during structured meals, such as lunch or dinner. Researchers believe that we imitate other people's food choices because we feel connected to them or want to like them. This can help loved ones make the right choices in situations. Now that we know some of the factors that influence our choices, we can take steps to take control of our eating habits. There are a few steps to get started. "Normal" is just a setting on your dryer.

This is an old saying that is still used today. Just because we think "everyone else is doing it" doesn't mean we should.

Delay.
Before choosing a food, stop for a moment and ask yourself if you are selecting that food because it aligns with your goals or because someone else is eating it.

Surround yourself with healthy choices. If your meal consists of a veggie and shrimp cocktail, your snack is less likely to be a cookie or some other snack that you and your friend accidentally nibbled at the same time.

Own the "why".
Other people in your social circle may not have the same goals as you, and that's okay! Wear something daily that reminds you why your health goals are essential.

be a positive influence on others.

Your healthy choices can support someone else's health goals.
As social beings, we are constantly influenced by others.
Knowing how our social context influences our behavior allows
us to make better choices that support our goals.

Creating a supportive environment

We know there is a stigma around obesity that needs to be
changed. But what should I do?
This is a complex issue that requires everyone's participation.
Creating a positive community environment is a step in the right
direction by focusing on what can be done to improve each
individual's overall health and well-being.

Invest in green space.

Introducing better and safer shared spaces allows people to use
the space instead of leaving it alone.
For example, accessible fitness equipment, water fountains and
seating are just some things that can be changed to create
inclusive green spaces. More spaces where people can exercise
safely, with interest and without judgment will have a positive
impact.

nutrition

Better labelling of packaged foods and more information on
preparing and cooking healthy foods are essential. Learning to

eat should start at a very early age, and educating children should no longer be left to parents. Schools must participate. As new health-related information continues to emerge, schools are ideal for education because they can be integrated into existing classrooms.

Promotion of junk food

We need to find ways to change junk food and drink advertising. Reporting calorie intake on a label is a step, but many people, especially children, still need to understand the data. The government recommends limiting the sale of junk food to children on all media platforms.

CHAPTER 8

Sedentary Lifestyle

A sedentary lifestyle occurs when you spend more than six hours a day sitting or lying down and do not engage in significant physical activity in your daily life.

This may sound familiar. For example, in office jobs, many people sit in front of a computer all day and then relax in front of the TV or phone before bed. It's easy, but with risks.

It may seem hard to believe that a sedentary lifestyle can cause health problems, but it is true. It can cause high blood pressure, weight gain, and other dangerous health problems. You may be drifting towards an increasingly sedentary lifestyle without realizing it. But there is always time to make changes that improve your health and well-being. Even the most minor changes to your daily routine can quickly make you more active.

Signs you may be sedentary

The symptoms of a sedentary lifestyle can manifest both physically and mentally and are sometimes so subtle that you don't even realize it's happening to you. It's essential to understand and recognize your symptoms so you can make adjustments to improve your health and quality of life. Signs of a sedentary lifestyle include:

• **Insomnia** – If you don't exercise much during the day, your body may not get the rest and recharge it needs at night, leading to sleep problems. Moderate exercise can help relieve mild fatigue, leading to better sleep.

• **Fatigue** – Not getting enough sleep at night can tell you how tired you are, but being sedentary can also be a significant factor. When you're active, your body releases endorphins, a burst of energy that improves your mood and relieves pain. May cause în.

• **Difficulty concentrating** – Have you noticed that your brain feels a little foggy or that you can't focus on tasks as much as you used to? Not getting enough physical activity can affect your attention, focus and motivation.

• **Pain** – If your neck or back hurts more than usual when sitting at your desk, you may need to exercise more.

• **Weight Gain** – As you work more from home, you may notice that your clothes feel slightly tighter when you walk into the office. This is because if you lead a sedentary lifestyle, you won't burn as many calories, which can lead to some weight gain. The influence of the way of living and living State and life can severely impact your health, which can significantly affect your subsequent physical and mental health in the long term.

Problems related to veins

If you don't exercise enough, blood flow can slow down, which can cause venous problems. These include varicose and varicose veins, deep vein thrombosis (DVT), venous thrombosis (SVT) or veins of the body. DVT can be life-threatening when blood clots travel to the lungs and block blood flow. SVT does not cause severe complications like DVT, but it can still cause pain. Physical activity is the best way to maintain blood circulation and prevent vein problems.

heart disease

Lack of physical activity can cause heart disease. These can include cardiomyopathy, which affects how the heart pumps blood. Coronary artery disease reduces the flow of oxygen-rich blood to the heart. Many factors can cause this condition, but the main one can be a lack of exercise. high cholesterol Cholesterol, a fatty substance your body needs to build healthy cells, can affect sedentary behaviour. High-density lipoprotein (HDL) is considered "good cholesterol," which helps remove low-density lipoprotein (LDL), or "bad cholesterol," from the blood. Not getting enough exercise can raise your cholesterol. In other words, too much LDL and too little HDL can cause arteriosclerosis, vascular problems, etc. It can cause it.

Hypertension (high blood pressure)

High blood pressure is when blood is pumped too hard around the body, causing the heart to work too hard. If your heart works too hard, your blood vessels can weaken. Being more active can be an easy way to control your blood pressure. Diabetes Insulin regulates blood sugar levels and the body's metabolism, allowing the body to use sugar for energy. Sitting for long periods can cause changes in your body, leading to insulin resistance and type 2 diabetes. Type 2 diabetes is more common in older people but can also be diagnosed in children. There is no cure, but exercise, weight loss and a healthy diet can help you overcome it.

obesity

Sedentary behaviour means you exercise less and burn fewer calories. Adults and teenagers should get at least 2.5 hours of exercise per week to reduce the risk of heart disease. However, a recent study found that only one in five people get the training they need, which can lead to unintended weight gain and obesity.

some types of cancer

Sedentary behaviour can increase the risk of developing endometrial, ovarian, and other types of cancer. You can reduce your cancer risk by staying active and changing your eating habits.

Stress, anxiety and depression

Physical activity releases serotonin in the brain, which improves your mood. Less serotonin is produced without physical activity, which can reduce positive feelings and motivation. Lack of motivation can make mental health more difficult to manage. It can be a complex cycle to navigate, but there are steps you can take to improve your mental health and well-being.

How can you change your sedentary lifestyle?

It's always possible to make even the most minor changes in your daily life, whether at home or work. You'll soon be on the right track by adjusting how you move, how much you move, and even making everyday tasks more enjoyable.

How to change your lifestyle at home

Life at home may seem mundane, with cooking, cleaning and eating vegetables. How can you change your situation to add more activity to your daily life? Move your body more.
The exercises should be done outside the gym. Go for a short walk, stretch, take a free online exercise class, or even run up and down the stairs a few times. If you still need to exercise, start slowly and contact your doctor to develop an exercise plan.

Turn housework into exercise.

You will have to do it anyway, so why not use it to your advantage? Try folding laundry, dancing while mopping, or cleaning items you usually spend less time cleaning, like the floor. Lighting up your house and sweating is a win.

Increase your rest time.
Sitting on the couch is fine, but there are easy ways to squeeze some activity into your downtime. Try standing, moving around, or doing floor exercises while watching TV. If you're talking on the phone or reading a book, walk around the house or yard. Lie on the floor and play with your children or pets. Playing and fighting for a while burns extra calories. If necessary, get preventive treatment.

You may stay longer and longer. If you've recognized the signs of a sedentary lifestyle, making an appointment with your doctor for an evaluation or consultation may be helpful. This helps to detect and prevent it before health problems start.

How to implement lifestyle changes in the workplace.
Most of the time, sitting and working and looking at the screen can occur during your work, and if you make a small change in your daily life, it will help you get out of the way you sit and live. Change your workspace
Make your workspace more active wherever you work, and think about desk ergonomics first. A standing desk is a good starting point for standing. See you on the way.

If you don't need a screen, hold a meeting where you walk and talk around your office or building. Or, if you have a phone appointment, you can answer the phone as you walk. If you have a question for a colleague, take the time to visit their office instead of emailing them. This will help you move, and the personal connections will help improve your mood. Change your everyday life.

Park a little further than usual to increase your step count. Take the stairs instead of the elevator and take occasional walks indoors or outdoors during the day. If you work from home, walk before sitting at the computer or include some light exercise in your schedule.

What other lifestyle changes can help?
Remember to start slow and build momentum and consistency so that more exercise becomes a habit. If you've tried some of these changes and aren't feeling any progress, don't worry. Feeling down or overwhelmed is easy, but there's nothing wrong with asking for help. Here are some additional ways to get support while leading an active lifestyle: mental health care Taking care of your mental health is not always possible. Talking to a mental health professional can be very helpful. social programs
Some employers offer health and wellness programs to their employees, and you can access them for free.

Talk to a weight loss expert.

If you've overcome some challenges but still aren't seeing the desired results, consult a weight loss expert to find a personalized approach.

Part III: Practical Strategies for Weight Loss

CHAPTER 9

Balanced Nutrition

This means eating various foods in appropriate proportions and consuming adequate amounts of food and drink to achieve and maintain a healthy weight.

A balanced diet contains sufficient amounts of all the nutrients your body needs for growth, health, and disease prevention. In addition, a healthy, balanced diet provides the necessary energy requirements, protects against vitamin, mineral, and other nutrient deficiencies, and strengthens immunity.

What are the benefits of a balanced diet?
A balanced diet helps provide your body with all the nutrients it needs to maintain normal growth and restore function.

Benefits of a healthy diet for adults
A healthy diet strengthens your immune system, reduces the risk of type 2 diabetes, cardiovascular disease, and some types of cancer, maintains a healthy weight, and helps you recover faster after disease and injury.

The benefits of healthy nutrition for children.
 Adequate nutrition helps strengthen bones, supports brain development, strengthens immunity, and regulates growth functions.

People with special dietary needs or medical conditions should seek advice from their doctor or registered dietitian. Food groups are included in the diet.
To eat a healthy, balanced diet, you need to:

Eat at least five servings of various fruits and vegetables per day.

Main foods high in fiber are starchy foods such as potatoes, bread, rice, pasta, etc.

Contains milk or milk substitutes (e.g., soy milk drinks).
Eat beans, peas, fish, eggs, meat, and other proteins.

Choose unsaturated fats and spreads and eat them in moderation.
Drink plenty of water (at least 6 to 8 glasses a day)

If you eat foods and drinks high in fat, salt, or sugar, eat them often and in small portions. To get a variety of nutrients, choose various foods from the five major food groups.

Many people eat and drink too many calories, too much saturated fat, sugar, and salt, and eat too little fruit, vegetables, fatty fish, or fiber.

The role of macronutrients.
Macronutrients are nutrients that your body needs in large amounts, including fats, carbohydrates, and proteins. These are nutrients that provide energy and are often called "macro." Macronutrients are components of food that are necessary to maintain body systems and structures. As part of a healthy diet, you need all three macronutrients, so none of them should be excluded or severely limited.

How much protein do you need?
Protein is essential for a variety of body functions, including:
Organizational structure
hormonal system,
metabolic system,
transportation system,
Enzymes that regulate metabolism
Acid/base balance.

The amount of protein you need depends on your weight and how much you exercise. The official Dietary Reference Intake ratio recommendation is 0.36 grams of protein per kilogram of body weight. The average sedentary person should consume about 56 grams of protein per day. The average sedentary woman should consume about 46 grams per day.

The more you exercise, the more protein you can safely consume. It would be best if you aimed to get 10-35% of your daily calories from protein. Your body cannot store protein. Once the required amount is reached, the body converts the rest into energy or fat. After you meet your daily requirements, the remaining calories should be concentrated in carbohydrates and fats.

When it comes to protein, where it comes from matters. While processed meat may have a lot of protein, it also has saturated fats and other ingredients that are bad for you. If possible, protein should come from plants. Plant sources provide not only protein but also fiber and micronutrients. The best plant-based sources of protein include:

beans

LENTILS

NUTS

seed

whole grains

If you do eat animal protein, choose healthier options such as:

backyard birds

over

Seafood

egg

About three servings of dairy products a day, especially yogurt

How many carbs do you need?

Carbohydrates fuel your body during intense exercise. They let your body use carbohydrates instead of proteins during exercise, which helps maintain muscle mass. In addition, carbohydrates offer energy for your central nervous system, including your brain. Carbohydrates are the most essential fuel for your body. You should get 45-65% of your calories from carbohydrates. As with protein, the type of food you get your carbs from is important. Carbohydrates are found in both healthy and unhealthy foods. The healthiest sources of carbohydrates can provide you with fiber, vitamins, minerals, and phytochemicals. Phytochemicals are compounds that help fight disease in plants. These include whole grains, legumes, vegetables, and fruits. Unhealthy sources of carbohydrates can raise blood sugar. It can cause weight gain, diabetes, and heart disease. These include foods that are easy to digest, such as white bread, pastries, soft drinks, and other highly processed foods.

How much fat do you need?

Fat is an integral part of your diet. Your body needs fat to:
Essential fatty acids that our bodies cannot produce
components of the cell wall
the energy source
Absorbs fat-soluble vitamins, including vitamins K, E, D, and A.
It insulates the body and protects the organs.

Aim to get 20-35% of your daily calories from fat. As with other macronutrients, it's essential to consume fats from healthy sources. The healthiest types of fats come from plants and are called monounsaturated and polyunsaturated fats. Good sources of these oils include:

olives and olive oil

rapeseed oil

peanut butter

avocado

nuts and nut butter

corn oil

sunflower oil

soybean oil

Saturated fats come mainly from animal and tropical oils and should not exceed 7-10% of your diet because they are linked to bad cholesterol and internal inflammation. Sources of saturated fat include:

Run Bliss

Warkensbliss

RUN

Calps Wells

High-fat dairy products

Processed meats such as hot dogs

Bonaire

Processed bakery products such as snacks

coconut and palm oil

Trans fats should be avoided as they increase bad cholesterol and lower good cholesterol. Cholesterol comes only from animal products. If your cholesterol is normal, you should consume less than 300g of cholesterol per day. If you have high cholesterol, limit your meal intake to less than 200 grams.

What is the difference between macronutrients and micronutrients?

Your body needs large amounts of macronutrients to function. Once you start reducing your intake, you can expect to lose weight. This can be difficult at first. This is especially true if you consistently control portion sizes at each meal. However, after a few weeks, you will start to see results, and it is gratifying. Of course, it will help to eat fewer high-calorie foods to lose weight regularly.

Five tips to control your portion sizes whenever you eat out or at home.

1. Top with lots of colorful vegetables.

This is the primary and most important way to control portion sizes. Eating more vegetables can help you lose weight and improve your overall nutrition. Plus, you don't have to compromise your bowel habits, skin health, or hair health while losing weight. Make sure at least 50% of your plate is filled with vegetables. The more color on the plate, the better the antioxidants, flavonoids, and polyphenols. Remember to include it in your meals, too. It could be as simple as hummus or guacamole or veggie sticks with cottage cheese instead of smoke and mayo. Starting small can go a long way in your fitness journey.

2. Eat before you get too hungry.

The main reason why someone overeats is a lack of discipline. It's always a good idea to be disciplined regarding mealtimes and general schedules. Our biological clock, our circadian rhythm, works best with a schedule. We are usually hungry at the same time every day, but due to work meetings or other reasons, we cannot eat on time.

When we realize we are hungry, we sit down and eat. We're probably starving. Low blood sugar combined with dehydration quickly removes plaque. Before we know it, we'll be overeating. The guilt factor then kicks in and signals the body to store more fat, which becomes a vicious cycle that needs to be broken. The best way to combat this is to eat before you get too hungry. Instead of eating after the session, eat before the lunch meeting. If you need to improve your understanding of your body's signals, stick to meal times. Additionally, eating slowly and taking more time to finish your meals are simple but practical ways to cut down on large portions.

3. Do not eat directly from the bag or box.

Do you have a habit of eating food directly from a bag, bag, or box? If so, this may be the biggest reason why you overeat at meal times. This is especially true if you watch or work while eating. People eat 50% more when given no visual cues about how much to eat. Therefore, if you cannot do without your favorite chips or cookies, divide their contents into small portions in advance (for example, from 5 to 10). If you are hungry or bored, you will eat directly from the bag or box rather than the whole portion.

4. Browse the buffet.

If you are a person who eats buffets as part of your job profile and portion control is your biggest struggle in such situations, we have a simple but practical tip for you. Examine and test each dish you serve in the buffet before serving the food. People often fill two-thirds of their plates with the first three dishes they see at the buffet. This can happen regardless of how healthy or unhealthy these foods are.

That's why going to the last food option on the buffet can help you make conscious choices about the foods you like and prevent you from eating foods you don't like or want to avoid.

5. Limit entertainment while eating.

Turn off the TV, stop working, and put your smartphone away while you eat. People who use their phones while eating eat more calories. Also, avoid using your lunch break for work. People feel less full when they eat while working on the computer.

6. Eat slowly

Taking your time when eating increases your enjoyment and reduces the amount of food you eat. For example, dim lighting and relaxing music create a relaxed dining atmosphere. Chew slowly, put your fork down between each bite, and drink water to extend your meal time.

7. Drink a glass of water.

It is recommended to drink 16 ounces (a large glass) of water before a meal. Filling your stomach with water reduces the chances of overeating. In addition, some symptoms of dehydration can cause hunger. Drink water when you are hungry. Thirst is often mistaken for hunger, so drinking water before a meal can help keep hunger at bay.

8. Use a small plate.

An easy way to control the amount of food you put on your plate is to use smaller plates. Smaller plates, knives, forks, glasses, and other utensils can help you eat less. Eliminating larger portions from your diet can reduce your energy intake by up to 29%.

9. Meal timing

The timing of meals is as important to your health as the ingredients and ingredients of the food. Consider different approaches to meeting proper meal times and improving your health. Let's discuss scientifically proven eating habits and strategies.

• Alternate meals and snacks at certain times of the day to control your calorie needs and hunger. Ideally, you should have three meals and two snacks a day. • Eat meals and snacks within 12 hours of each day. The most suitable 12-hour period is between 6:00 a.m. and 6:00 p.m. • Eat more calories at meals throughout the day, including breakfast, brunch, and lunch. Dinner and supper should be low in calories. • Eat whole foods and nutritious snacks instead of processed or packaged foods that contain significant amounts of sugar and fat.

• Depending on your goals, you can consider various approaches, including gaining, maintaining, or losing weight. For example, intermittent fasting is a scientifically proven approach to treating obesity, diabetes, and heart disease.

Research shows that ideal meal times are:
Eat a breakfast rich in protein and calories. The best time is 7 a.m., within 30 minutes of waking up.

Eat a high-calorie lunch 4 hours after breakfast. The best time is from 13:00 to 16:00.

Dinner should be half your lunch, ideally around 7 p.m. Eat dinner 3 hours before bed.

Between meals, eat light snacks based on natural foods. The benefits of consuming food at the right time

Maintain a good routine.
Eating at regular times helps you maintain good habits. You will feel less stressed calmer, sleep well on time, and wake up on time for work. Improved digestion
Eating regularly gives the digestive tract enough time to digest and absorb food and nutrients properly.

Decrease in fat storage.
Regular mealtimes help reduce body fat accumulation. Eating five small meals instead of two or three large meals causes your body to use more dietary fat for energy, which reduces fat storage.

Should I eat right before bed?
Eating before bed is not a healthy habit because of the following effects:

• Sleep disturbances depending on the type of food consumed

• Acid reflux causes heartburn due to the horizontal position of the body during sleep

• Lower your body's metabolic rate, which can lead to slower digestion and weight gain

• Stomach pain is also common in people who eat a lot before going to bed

CHAPTER 10

Effective Exercise

There is no magic way to exercise. You get out what you put in. That doesn't mean you have to practice for hours every day. It just means you have to work with your heart.

Not all exercises are created equal. Some are more effective than others, targeting multiple muscle groups, suitable for different fitness levels, or helping you burn calories more efficiently.

So what is the best exercise?

1. Walking

Any exercise program should include cardiovascular exercises that strengthen your heart and burn calories. And walking is an exercise that can be done anywhere, anytime, with no equipment other than good shoes.

It is not suitable for beginners either. Even fit people can exercise by walking. Brisk walking can burn up to 500 calories per hour. It takes 3,500 calories to lose a pound, so if you do nothing, you can expect to lose a pound every seven hours of walking. Walking off the couch for an hour a day isn't enough, but if you're a beginner, it's a good idea to start by walking for 5 to 10 minutes at a time and gradually work your way up to at least 30 minutes per session.

Only add up to 5 minutes at a time. Another tip: It's best to increase your walking time before increasing your speed or incline.

2. interval training

Whether you're a beginner or veteran, hiker or aerobic dancer, adding interval training to your cardio will improve your fitness and help you lose weight.

Varying the pace during exercise promotes adaptation of the aerobic system. The stronger your aerobic system, the more calories you can burn.

The way to do this is to increase the intensity or speed for 1 to 2 minutes, then rest for 2 to 10 minutes (depending on your total exercise time and how much time you need to recover).

Continue this throughout your workout.

3. Squats

Strength training is vital. The more muscle you have, the more calories you can burn.

Experts prefer strength training that targets multiple muscle groups. Squats, which work your quadriceps, hamstrings, and glutes, are a good example.

It gives you the most benefit because it works for several muscle groups simultaneously. But form is fundamental.

What makes an exercise functional is how it is performed. If your technique is good, it will work.

For perfect form, keep your feet shoulder-width apart and your back straight. Bend your knees and lower your hips. Your knees should be as high as your ankles.

Even if you think you are sitting on a chair, there is no chair, It can be helpful to practice with an actual chair. Start by getting in and out of the actual seat properly. Once you get used to it, hit your bum on the chair and stand up again. Then, perform the same movements without the chair.

Many patients complain of knee pain due to weakness of the quadriceps muscles. If you experience pain when climbing stairs, strengthening your quads with squats can be very helpful.

4. Lunges

Like squats, lunges work all the major muscles of the lower body: glutes, quads, and hamstrings.

Lunges are a great exercise because they mimic life. It's like walking, only exaggerated. Lunges are a more advanced exercise than squats and help improve your balance.

Here's how to do it right: Take significant steps and keep your spine neutral. Bend your front knee to about a 90-degree angle, keeping your weight on your back toes and focusing on bringing the knee of your back leg into the floor.

Petersen suggests imagining yourself standing on your hind legs. The back leg is the leg you should be standing on.

For a more functional run, you can go backward and sideways as well as forward. The better you prepare yourself to assume different positions throughout the day, the more beneficial your exercise will be.

5. push-ups

When done correctly, push-ups instantly strengthen your chest, shoulders, triceps, and core muscles.

Push-ups can be done at any fitness level. For beginners, start pushing up at counter height. Then bend your knees and place your toes on the floor, then on a table, chair, or floor."

Here's how to do the perfect push-ups:

1. Place your hands slightly wider than shoulder-width apart and face down.
2. Place your toes or knees on the floor and keep your body in a perfect diagonal from your shoulders to your knees or feet.
3. Train your glutes [back muscles] and abdominal muscles.
4. Bend and straighten your elbows, lowering and raising your body, keeping your body stable at all times.

6. Abdominal Crunches

Who doesn't want toned and toned abs? When done right, known spells (including variants) are good choices for target selection.

For a standard stretch, start by lying on your back with your feet on the floor and your head resting on your toes. Begin the exercise by pressing your lower back down and contracting your abdominal muscles, first lifting your head (after tucking your chin in slightly) and then lifting your neck, shoulders, and upper back off the floor.

Don't stick your chin out or pull your neck forward. Hold your breath and keep your elbows out of sight to keep your chest and shoulders open. Do the exercise with your feet on the floor and your knees bent. Many people who keep their feet on the ground tend to arch their backs and contract their hip flexors. Crunches can be great, but if done incorrectly, they can arch your back and weaken your abs.

To exercise your obliques (lower back muscles), grab a standard bench press and twist on the floor, rotating your spine to one side. Turn back before they come. It is crucial to change direction first. Because it's the slope that lifts you, but remember that crunches alone won't give you a flat stomach. Burning belly fat requires the well-known formula of eating more calories than you burn. Crunches train your abdominal muscles. Please don't confuse them with abdominal exercises to burn fat. This is the biggest myth in sports.

7. Bent over Row

Talk about a bang for the money; this exercise works all the major back muscles and the biceps. Here's how to do it with good form: Stand with your feet shoulder-width apart, knees bent, and hips forward. (If this exercise is challenging to do standing, try sitting on an incline bench and lifting your weight back.) Lean your hips forward slightly, tighten your abdominal muscles, and extend your upper back for support. Hold dumbbells or barbells under your shoulders with your hands shoulder-width apart. Bend your elbows and raise your hands to the sides. Pause briefly and slowly lower your arms to return to the starting position. (Beginners should perform the movements without weights.)

Creating an exercise routine.

Starting a fitness program can be one of the best things you can do for your health. Physical activity can reduce the risk of chronic disease, improve balance and coordination, aid in weight loss, and improve sleep habits and self-esteem. And there is even better news. You can start your fitness program in just five steps.

1. Assess your fitness level

You probably know how fit you are. However, assessing and recording your baseline fitness score can give you a gauge to measure your progress. To assess your aerobic and strength training, flexibility, and body composition, consider the following:

Heart rate before and after running a mile

This is the time it takes to walk 1 mile or run 1.5 miles (2.41 km).

How many standard or modified push-ups can you do at once?

The ability to sit on the floor and stretch your legs forward

Waist circumference, just above the hip bone, your body mass index

2. Create your fitness program

It's easy to say you exercise every day. But it would help if you had a plan. When designing your fitness program, consider the following:

Think about your fitness goals. Starting a fitness program to lose weight? Or do you have other motivations, like training for a marathon? Having specific goals helps you measure your progress and stay motivated. Create a balanced work routine. Do at least 150 minutes per week of moderate aerobic activity, 75 minutes of vigorous aerobic activity, or a combination of moderate and vigorous activity. The guidelines recommend doing this exercise for one week. It is recommended that you exercise at least 300 minutes per week for more excellent health benefits and to help you lose or maintain weight. However, even a little physical activity is beneficial. Being active for short periods during the day has health benefits. Do strength training for all major muscle groups at least twice a week. Try to perform one set of each exercise with a weight or resistance level that fatigues your muscles after about 12 to 15 repetitions. Start low and grow slowly. If you are new to exercise, start slow and build up slowly. If you have an injury or illness, consult your doctor or exercise therapist to help you develop a fitness program that gradually improves your range of motion, strength, and endurance.

Incorporate activity into your daily life. Finding time to exercise can be difficult. To make things easier, plan your training time like you would any other meeting. Watch your favorite show while walking on the treadmill, study on a stationary bike, or relax by walking to work.

We plan to include a variety of activities. Varied activities (cross-training) can help keep your workouts from getting boring. Low-impact cross-training, such as cycling or aquatic exercise, also reduces the risk of injury or strain to specific muscles or joints. Plan alternate exercises emphasizing different body parts, such as walking, swimming, or strength training. Try high-intensity interval training. High-intensity interval training involves performing short bursts of high-intensity activity separated by recovery periods of lower-intensity activity.

Give yourself time to recover. Many people start with a frenzy that is too long or intense and give up when their muscles and joints become sore or injured. Plan time for the body to rest and recover between sessions. Please write it down on paper. A written plan will motivate you to stay on track.

3. Gather your equipment

Let's start with sneakers. Choose the proper footwear for the activity you have in mind. For example, athletic shoes are lighter and offer more support than cross-training shoes. If you invest in fitness equipment, choose something practical, comfortable, and easy to use. You can try out some equipment at a fitness center before investing in your equipment. We recommend using a fitness app for your smart device or another activity tracker that tracks distance, calories burned, or heart rate.

4. start working

Now, you are ready to act. When starting a fitness program, keep the following in mind:

Start slow and build up gradually. Allow plenty of time to warm and cool down by simply walking or stretching. Then, increase the speed to a pace you can maintain for 5 to 10 minutes without getting too tired. As endurance improves, gradually increase training time. Exercise for 30 to 60 minutes most days of the week. Disassemble the item if necessary. You don't have to do all the exercises simultaneously so you can stay active throughout the day. You can also get aerobic benefits by doing shorter but more frequent sessions. Training in short sessions several times daily may fit your schedule better than a 30-minute session. Any amount of activity is better than no activity.

Be creative. Exercise can include various activities, including walking, cycling, and rowing. But don't stop there. Enjoy a weekend family outing or an evening of ballroom dancing. Find activities you enjoy that you can add to your fitness routine.

Listen to your body. Rest if you feel pain, shortness of breath, dizziness, or nausea. You might be pushing yourself too hard.

Sensitivity. If you're not feeling well, take a day or two off.

5. Track your progress

Repeat your fitness assessment six weeks after starting the program and every few months afterward. You may need to increase your practice time to continue making progress. Or, you might be surprised you're getting just the right amount of exercise to reach your fitness goals.

If you feel unmotivated, try setting a new goal or trying a new activity. It can also help to exercise with a friend or take a class at a fitness center.

Starting an exercise program is a big decision. But there shouldn't be too many. With careful planning and setting your own pace, you can develop healthy habits that will last a lifetime.

Maximize your calorie burn.

While you can burn calories during aerobic exercise, strength training is a low-calorie burner that keeps your metabolism revving long after you stop exercising.

During intense exercise, the oxygen level in the body is lower than usual, e.g., Hypoxia) causes the body to consume more oxygen after exercise, causing you to burn 6 to 15% more

calories the rest of the day and night. In addition, improving metabolism has positive health effects beyond burning calories, including lowering blood pressure and improving cardiovascular health. HIIT (High Intensity Interval Training)
Studies have shown that 27-minute high-intensity interval training (HIIT) sessions three times a week provide the same anaerobic and aerobic exercise benefits as 60-minute cardio sessions five times a week. Less time, same results! Most of Seven's workouts are HIIT workouts.

Watch your form.
By tensing your muscles and maintaining a solid core during each exercise, you can continue to burn calories efficiently during your session. Do you like to run? Proper technique will increase your speed, allowing you to cover greater distances in less time and burn up to 15% more calories.

Add a beat.
Creating a great playlist to listen to during your workout can help you burn more calories and extend your workout time by 20%. Music has been shown to help athletes ignore signs of fatigue, get into the zone, and maintain a fast pace by synchronizing movements to the beat.

Find a workout buddy.
Having a workout buddy has been shown to help you stick to your workouts, exercise more, and reach your goals faster.

Add more weight

Using heavier weights and lower repetitions is a great way to burn more calories during strength training. That's because heavy weights promote the breakdown of protein in the muscles, forcing the body to use more energy to repair itself.

CHAPTER 11

Behavioral Change

Behavioral change can be a temporary or permanent effect, considered a change in an individual's behavior compared to previous behavior. Changes in thinking, interpretation, feelings, or relationships usually characterize these changes. Behavior change refers to long-term changes in habits and behavior. Many studies on health behavior show that small changes can dramatically improve people's health and life expectancy. These changes may adversely affect the health of other people.

Examples include:

quit smoking

Reduce your alcohol consumption

healthy food

Exercise regularly

Practice safe sex

stay safe

How to get started.

Whether people want to lose weight, quit smoking, or achieve another goal, one solution may only fit some. Achieving your goals may require trial and error. This is when many people give up on their behavior change goals. The key to achieving and maintaining your goals is to try new methods and find ways to stay motivated. Change may not come quickly, but psychologists have discovered effective ways to help people change their behavior. These techniques are used by therapists, doctors, and teachers. Understanding the elements of change, the stages, and how to progress through each stage will help you achieve your goals.

Elements of change.

To be successful, you need to understand the three most essential elements of behavior change.

• Readiness for change: Do you have the resources and knowledge to implement sustainable change successfully?

• Barriers to change: Are there factors that prevent change?

• Risk of relapse: What factors can lead to a relapse of the previous behavior?

Set Realistic goals.

Setting realistic goals benefits everyone. No one knows the future and how our needs and aspirations may change over time. Adaptability teaches us not to abandon our plans when circumstances change. In a world full of uncertainty, adaptation is essential.

Specific goals are flexible and adaptable. Revising our action plan and adapting to new situations will help us achieve our goals. When things don't go as planned, you can rely on persistence, willpower, hope, and the ability to deal with uncertainty to get you through. If you are optimistic about them, they are more likely to achieve their goals. Maintaining a growth mindset will set you up for success. Some people wonder why their goals have to be realistic and then become frustrated when they don't achieve them in the desired time frame. A vivid example of this is New Year's resolutions. If someone hopes to lose 10 pounds, learn Spanish, get a promotion, or become a vegetarian, they ask too much of themselves.

It's easy to understand why people get frustrated and give up. Focus on developing small habits and skills that can help you achieve bigger goals, for example, creating an exercise routine, enrolling in a beginner's Spanish course, or working to become a better leader.

Unattainable goals often end in failure, which can lead to a lot of self-critical thinking and low self-esteem. Continuing to set unattainable goals can cause people to give up rather than try to adapt to change. But if you have manageable goals, you can focus your time and energy on achievable things. Trackable goals and achievements reinforce our positive emotions and motivate us to set new goals. Keeps optimism high and boosts self-esteem. These unrealistic goals happen when we don't plan our lives and don't think automatically. It is crucial to have a plan to achieve your goals.

How to set realistic goals.

Learning how to set and achieve goals may seem simple, but there is more to it than memorizing goals. If you're having trouble setting long-term goals right now, take a step back and think about specific goals you can achieve right now that will help you get there.

Check out these 11 tips to help you learn how to set achievable goals.

1. Consider which organizational model is best for you.

2. Think about how you will measure your goals.

Three. Have confidence in yourself and your abilities

4. Set SMART goals

5. Include your goals in future plans

6. Gather the resources and tools you need to succeed.

7. Remember to adjust your goals if necessary.

8. Align your goals with your life values.

9. Let us know when you want to check on our progress.

10. Set a realistic time frame to achieve your goal.

11. Ensure your progress by creating a vision board or visualizing your dream future.

Ten examples of specific objectives.

Specific goals come in all shapes and sizes. This can include work goals, personal goals, and everything in between. Your goals can be collaborative with others, but they can also be very personal. No matter where you aim, you must have a clear plan and specific goals.

To help you start thinking, here are ten examples of realistic goals:

1. Set boundaries with your peers

2. Practice your time management skills

Three. Make more time for your mental health

4. Learn new skills to get promoted

5. Support your community food bank

6. Develop a new social media optimization strategy for your business.

7. Improve your graphic design skills

8. Encourage team members to work more collaboratively.

9. Take complete control of your financial budget each month

10. Improve your communication skills in professional and personal settings.

Overcoming Plateaus and Staying Motivated.

Starting your fitness journey can be fun and rewarding, but it's not uncommon to hit plateaus along the way. A plateau is when progress seems to stop, and motivation begins to wane. However, it is important to remember that plateaus are a natural part of any fitness endeavor and provide growth opportunities. In this blog post, we'll cover some practical strategies and tips to help you stay motivated and push through plateaus during your KILLER workout. Let's jump in!

Assessment and focus.

The first step when experiencing a plateau is to assess your current exercise routine and goals. Take a moment to reflect on your journey so far and objectively assess your progress. Ask yourself if your goals still match your current desires and if you need to adjust your exercise or diet, such as reducing your calorie intake to create a healthy deficit to gain or regain the weight you lost to new energy development. This self-reflection will help you refocus your efforts and set new goals if necessary.

Improve your exercise routine.

A common reason for plateaus is that the exercise is too comfortable. The body adapts to the same exercise over time, resulting in poor performance. To overcome this problem, strengthen by lifting heavier weights, challenging yourself to perform more reps, or taking the technique to the next level (e.g., push-ups to knee-to-leg push-ups). By challenging yourself frequently during your training, you can break plateaus and make further progress.

Set SMART goals.

Setting specific, measurable, achievable, relevant, and time-bound (SMART) goals is essential to stay motivated during plateaus. Break down your overall fitness goals into smaller, more manageable steps. For example, if your goal is to lose weight, focus on losing a certain amount of weight per week or gradually increasing the amount of exercise you do. At 9Round, we recommend starting with at least three weekly workouts and building up gradually. Hitting these small milestones can give you a sense of accomplishment and motivate you to push through plateaus.

Track your progress.

Monitoring progress is important to stay motivated. Fortunately, the 9Round PULSE makes it easy to track your workouts with its heart rate system. Your online subscription portal keeps a record of every workout you complete. This includes the number of calories you've burned, the number of PULSE points you've earned, and your average heart rate during your workout. Also, consider tracking other metrics like body measurements, body fat percentage, and mood during exercise. Progress tracking lets you see how far you've come, even when the scale isn't moving. This tangible proof of progress will re-energize your motivation and give you the boost you need to overcome plateaus.

Ask a champion trainer for help.

If you are constantly struggling to overcome plateaus, seek professional guidance. Your Champion Trainer is ready to provide specific advice tailored to your specific training needs and goals. It helps you evaluate your current routine, identify areas for improvement, and introduce you to new ways to take your 9Round workouts to the next level. Plus, working closely with a champion trainer will help you stay motivated and give you the accountability and support you need to succeed on your fitness journey.

As you can see, plateaus are inevitable during your fitness journey, but they don't have to hinder your progress. By implementing these strategies and tips, you can overcome plateaus, re-motivate, and continue to reach your fitness goals.

With determination and perseverance, you will become stronger, stronger, and more motivated than ever. Dedicate yourself and succeed, and it will be yours!

CHAPTER 12

Mind and Body Wellness

A healthy body and a healthy mind go together. The two are much more connected than you might think, and when one fights, the other is negatively affected. Your body and mind work together to help you succeed in everyday life. Your thoughts can affect the way your body feels and behaves, and the way your body feels can affect your thoughts. This is called the mind-body connection and determines how the body responds to stress. Worrying and worrying about finances, work, family life, and other issues can lead to stress, which can lead to muscle tension, headaches, stomach problems, and more. These things often add up and become a vicious cycle that leads to mental exhaustion.

Improving your physical and mental well-being can have huge benefits, but many people need help knowing where to start.

The connection between mind and body

The health of the body and mind is important.

Well-being is not a passive state or something to be taken for granted, but something we must actively pursue through our intentions and actions. Many body systems work together to maintain good health and improve your health.

While illness, environmental factors, and injury are beyond our control, we can control our coping strategies and determine how quickly we bounce back from setbacks. One of the most effective things you can do is change the way you think—how the world affects you and how you affect yourself and yourself. This means recognizing that much of our life is determined by our physical, social, and cultural environment and taking responsibility for our thoughts, actions, and choices. Focusing on self-improvement and self-forgiveness are two of the best things you can do to improve your mind-body connection.

Stress management.
Stress is a constant factor in our lives. This is how our body responds to challenges and adapts to and overcomes threats. However, excessive stress can affect our mind and body. Stress management is the key to improving the health of the body. There are several ways to control stress:

• Respiratory exercise for rest

• Images aimed at rest

• the gradual relaxation of the muscles

• Yoga movement

• Make the body and mind comfortable

In addition to these exercises, you can also:

• Sleep more than 7 hours each evening.

• healthy and nourishing food

• Training formation

• Thank you every day

• Enjoy the walk and outdoors

• Use positive thinking

• Have time with friends

• Get a new hobby

There are many ways to improve physical health. Once you find a method that works for you, you'll find that your body and mind work more efficiently, and your stress levels decrease.

A holistic approach to weight loss.

Obesity in women.

The obesity pattern seen in women is usually pear-shaped obesity. Obese women are at high risk of developing various lifestyle diseases, including gallbladder cancer, breast cancer, uterine cancer, cervical cancer, and ovarian cancer. In addition, obesity can increase a woman's risk of obstetric and gynecological complications. These include infertility, menstrual disorders, miscarriage, and mother-child problems.

Obesity in men.

Because they are generally apple-shaped, men are at greater risk of abdominal obesity, which is an independent risk factor for heart disease and type 2 diabetes. Obesity in men has been linked to many other diseases, including erectile dysfunction! A holistic weight loss program involves not only helping you lose weight but also improving your overall well-being, including:

1. Find your body type and work for it.
2. Improved lifestyle and quality of life
Three. Improving resting metabolism
4. Improve indicators of physical condition and endurance
5. Improving health indicators
6. Preventing the risk of illness or complications
7. balanced body composition
8. Help me feel better
9. Lose or lose weight.

10. Improves sleep quality

Five ways to lose weight permanently
A practical and sustainable weight loss program should focus on five key areas:

1. Healthy lifestyle

The way we live affects our health. This is evident in many studies. A smart lifestyle can help you prevent disease, increase your sense of well-being, and build a leaner, stronger body. Diet, exercise, hydration, rest, and quality sleep are the most important lifestyle habits to focus on.

2. State of health

Obesity or weight gain can cause food allergies, diabetes, acute and chronic inflammation, and more. It can vary depending on several health problems, such as Being overweight, which indicates that there are too many toxins in our body. Therefore, it should be considered and corrected as the first step in losing weight.

3. Biochemical systems

Weight gain is a side effect of (almost all) antidepressants. Our body's hormones are influenced by food, exercise, sleep, stress, and more. It determines our reactions to external stimuli such as Hormones, plays a vital role in our body's metabolism, and can be disrupted by drugs. Fat accumulation and breakdown can be associated with up-or-down-regulation of the endocrine system. Another critical factor that determines our biochemical system is our genes.

4. holistic approach

A holistic approach to weight loss should focus on working at the bottom level to identify root causes contributing to weight gain or loss. This includes various aspects of diet and nutrition aimed at providing essential micronutrients, including quality macros, herbal remedies, natural supplements, adequate amounts of soluble and insoluble fiber, and adequate fluid intake. To complement this, it can be helpful to add yoga, breathing exercises, physical movement, and mindfulness exercises to your daily routine.

5. Clear Vision/Focus

People who are clear about their reasons for losing weight (whether it's something as simple as putting on a dress or a severe health issue) do better than those who think being thin is "fun." Instead of thinking about the process, desires, or challenges, focus on why you are doing this program. You will understand how easy it is to make the right choice.

Part IV:
Long-Term Success and Maintenance

CHAPTER 13

Building a Support System

Connecting with other people is vital for happiness, self-esteem, and coping. Even if you recognize the importance of a support system, it can be easier to build a network of healthy and supportive people.

A support system can help you manage stress and increase life satisfaction, meaning, and fulfillment. Support systems can include relationships with many people, including family, friends, coworkers, and classmates. You are unique in the type and number of relationships you want and the support you need.

What are the benefits of social support?

- Personal satisfaction
- To feel connected and cared for.
- Improved self-esteem
- Improved physical and mental health
- Stress reduction and resilience.

Types of personal support systems.

A support system consists of people who help, respect, and care. There are different types of personal support.

• Emotional Support System: These are non-judgmental people who always have your best interests in mind and give honest feedback.

• Professional Support System: Whether at school or work, these are the professional connections you need to help you achieve your goals.

• Social Support System: Even if you don't have close ties, these are connections with people in your community who have a positive impact on your life.

Tips for building a support system.
We all need people. So, how do you manage the hustle and bustle of modern life and create a healthy support system for your life? Here are some tips to help you get started:

1. Find out who the healthy Supports in your life are.
List people you know, including family, friends, advisors, and community acquaintances. Then ask yourself:

• Do they respect you?
• Do you trust them?
• Does it bring out the best in you?
• Does it help you feel happier and more positive?
If yes, then it's time to develop those relationships.

2. Build on existing bonds.

Some of the best sources of support already exist. Whether you've lost touch with a friend or a new relationship, there are easy ways to reconnect with existing friends.

- Stay in touch with phone calls, texts and emails.
- Tell these people how much they mean to you.
- Give your child a chance to vent during difficult times.
- Accept help when you need it.

3. Embrace common interests.

If you need to expand your support system, you're sure to have like-minded people around you. The best way to build relationships and friendships is through regular interaction. There are many ways to meet people in your community:

- Join a sports or sports team.
- voluntary.
- Join a hobby class or group.
- Start a book club.

4. Expand your professional connections.

If you are career-oriented, it may be a good idea to focus on your professional support network. These are people inside and outside the industry who can help you advance your career or give you advice. People considering other careers can help you understand and deal with work-related stress better than anyone else.

5. Get expert guidance.

Support may mean contacting a therapist, counselor, or addiction specialist if you need help. Having a qualified professional guide you through your struggles, help you identify your weaknesses, and serve as part of your personal support system can make a big difference.

Family, friends, and weight loss

Finding support for your weight loss efforts can mean the difference between success and failure. Build your team around these ideas.

If you don't have a weight loss support group, use these strategies to create one. If so, reach out to your team and let them know how important their support is to you. Research shows that having friends and family who support your healthy eating and exercise goals is critical to long-term weight loss success. Support may include:

• Emotional: A shoulder to lean on when you're feeling down.
• Practitioner: Someone to watch the children while they practice.

• Inspiration: Your workout partner who encourages you to get outside and exercise on those days when your favorite show feels better.

Tell your family and friends that you appreciate their help, and be specific about how they can help you. For example, you could ask your partner to go with you and have your best friend with you when you need an answer.
You can expect unaccepted behavior. It's no surprise that losing weight puts you at risk for your partner or spouse. If you don't try her famous dessert, your mom might get sick, or your friends might ask you to skip your workout and go out for pizza. Remind them that changing their lifestyle won't change how they feel about their loved ones. Offer specific ways to help you achieve your goals and share your journey.

Find support.
Having a solid support system can encourage and motivate you. Support systems come in all forms and are great resources for sharing and learning from each other. These may include women-only services, men-only services, faith-based services, services provided in local community centers, or services provided online. Finding a support system doesn't have to be complicated!
Here are five ways to support your weight loss journey:

1. Local fitness group

A local fitness group allows you to work out with others and build camaraderie while working out. Some are offered at local gyms, while others are offered at local community centers. Exercising in a group setting can help you stay confident and motivated even in the worst times.

2. Private groups to help you lose weight

A private weight loss support group is no different than joining a support group for a specific condition, such as diabetes or polycystic ovary syndrome (PCOS). These groups can help you openly discuss your problems and overcome unhealthy behaviors with healthy people. They provide camaraderie as well as support and accountability. Where can I find it? Check local messages and community forums, or ask your doctor.

3. Social Networks and Applications

If in-person support isn't your thing, social media and apps are good options. Most health-based apps offer behavior change tools such as calorie trackers, nutrition labeling tips, exercise logs, and digital food diaries. Most have forums where you can chat with others and get advice. Social media groups and communities also allow you to connect with others with similar interests and share weekly health tips and motivations. You can find many of these groups by searching for hashtags based on your interests, such as #plant-based, #yogalifestyle, #homeworkout, #nutritiontips, or #weightlossmotivation.

4. Commercial programs

Commercial programs may cost more because they are paid services, but they can provide a personalized, structured plan to help you reach your weight goals. Some programs help participants stay motivated and focused. Many of these programs come with online communities and virtual health coaches to keep you inspired and accountable. This is a good option if you are okay with paying extra for a weight loss plan that fits your needs.

5. medical worker

To help you lose weight, you may need more professional support than family or friends. There are many healthcare providers with specialized training, from behavioral therapists and psychologists to nutritionists and physicians. If you are struggling with issues such as eating disorders, depression, anxiety, chronic stress, or substance abuse, you may want to consider seeking professional counseling.

CHAPTER 14

Weight Maintenance Strategies

Unfortunately, many people who lose weight end up gaining it back.

Only about 20% of people who start dieting while overweight manage to lose weight and keep it off long-term. But don't let that discourage you. From exercise to stress management, there are several scientifically proven ways to lose weight.

Why do people gain weight again?

There are several common reasons why people regain the weight they have lost. This is often associated with unrealistic expectations and feelings of deprivation.

• Restricted diet: Extreme calorie restriction can slow your metabolism and alter your appetite-regulating hormones, contributing to weight gain.

• Myth: If you think of dieting as a quick fix rather than a long-term health solution, you're more likely to give up and regain the weight you've lost.

• Lack of consistent habits: Most diets are based on willpower rather than habits you can incorporate into your daily life. They focus on rules rather than lifestyle changes, which prevents weight loss.

Many diets are too restrictive, with requirements that are difficult to follow. Additionally, many people need to have the right mindset before starting a diet, which can lead to weight gain.

1. Exercise often

Regular exercise plays a vital role in maintaining weight. This will help you burn extra calories and increase your metabolism. These are two necessary elements to achieve energy balance. Being in energy balance means you burn the same number of calories as you expend. As a result, your weight stays the same. Several studies have shown that people who do at least 200 minutes per week (30 minutes per day) of moderate physical activity after losing weight are more likely to maintain their weight loss. In some cases, much higher physical activity levels may be required to maintain weight successfully. One review concluded that one hour of exercise per day is optimal for people trying to lose weight. It's important to remember that exercise is most beneficial for weight maintenance when combined with other lifestyle changes, including a healthy diet. Exercising for at least 30 minutes daily can help you maintain weight by balancing calorie intake and expenditure.

2. Try to eat breakfast every day

Eating breakfast can help you achieve your weight loss goals. People who eat breakfast tend to have healthy habits, such as exercising more and consuming more fiber and micronutrients. Additionally, eating breakfast is one of the most common behaviors reported by people who have successfully lost weight. One study found that of 2,959 people who lost 30 pounds in at least a year, 78 percent reported eating breakfast daily. Breakfast eaters have great success in losing weight, but the evidence is mixed. Studies have not shown that skipping breakfast automatically leads to weight gain or nutritional deficiencies.

Skipping breakfast can help some people achieve their weight loss and maintenance goals. It can be one of the things that affect a person's personality.

If you think breakfast will help you reach your goals, you should eat breakfast. But if you don't like breakfast or you're not hungry in the morning, it's okay to skip it.

People who eat breakfast develop healthy habits that help them maintain their weight. However, skipping breakfast does not automatically lead to weight gain.

3. Eat more protein

Eating more protein can help you maintain your weight because protein helps reduce appetite and increase satiety.

Protein causes satiety and increases the levels of certain hormones in the body that are important for weight management. Protein also reduces the level of hormones that increase hunger.

Protein's effects on hormones and satiety can automatically reduce the calories you eat each day, which are essential factors in weight maintenance. In addition, it takes a significant amount of energy for the body to break down. Therefore, regular consumption increases the calories you burn during the day. The impact of protein on metabolism and appetite is most noticeable when about 30% of calories are consumed from protein. That's 150 grams of protein in a 2,000-calorie diet.

Protein helps maintain weight by promoting satiety, increasing metabolism, and reducing total calorie intake.

4. Measure yourself regularly

Getting on the scale regularly and checking your weight can be a valuable tool in maintaining your weight. It tells you your progress and encourages your weight management efforts. People who weigh themselves may eat fewer calories throughout the day, which can help them lose weight. One study found that people who weighed themselves six days a week ate an average of 300 fewer calories per day than those who weighed themselves less often.

How often you weigh yourself is a personal choice. Some people find it helpful to weigh themselves every day, while others find it helpful to check their weight once or twice a week.

Weighing yourself can help you maintain weight by monitoring your progress and actions.

5. Consider your carbohydrate intake

Paying attention to the types and amounts of carbohydrates you eat will make weight loss easier. Eating too many refined carbohydrates, such as white bread, white pasta, and fruit juice, can harm your weight maintenance goals.

These foods have been stripped of their natural fibers, essential to ensure fullness. Diets low in fiber are associated with weight gain and obesity.

Limiting total carbohydrate intake can help maintain weight loss. Studies have shown that people who follow low-carb diets sometimes maintain their weight loss long-term after losing it. In addition, people on low-carb diets tend to consume more calories than they need to burn to maintain weight.

Limiting your intake of carbohydrates, especially refined carbohydrates, can help prevent weight gain.

6. Lifting weights

Loss of muscle mass is a common side effect of weight loss. Losing muscle can limit your ability to maintain weight because your metabolism slows down, and you burn fewer calories throughout the day.

Doing some type of resistance exercise, such as lifting weights, can help prevent muscle loss and, in turn, maintain or improve your metabolism. Studies have shown that people who gain weight after losing weight maintain their weight by maintaining muscle mass.

To get these benefits, we recommend strength training at least twice a week. Exercise therapy should train all muscle groups for optimal results.

Lifting weights at least twice a week can help you maintain your weight by maintaining muscle mass, which is essential for a healthy metabolism.

7. Prepare for failure

When you maintain your weight, failure is inevitable. You may find yourself giving in to unhealthy cravings or giving up on exercise.

But just because you make the occasional mistake doesn't mean you have to overshoot your goals. Keep making good choices. It also helps you plan for situations where healthy eating can be difficult, such as upcoming holidays or vacations. After losing weight, you may experience a setback or two. If you plan and start right away, you can overcome challenges.

8. Stick to a schedule all week (even on weekends).

A habit that often leads to weight gain is eating healthy during the week and cheating on the weekend. This mindset can often lead people to eat junk food, which can set back their efforts to maintain weight.

If this becomes a regular habit, you may gain more weight than you initially lost. Studies show that people who follow a consistent diet throughout the week are more likely to lose weight in the long term.

One study found that people who were consistent each week were almost twice as likely to lose 5 pounds per year compared to those who allowed more flexibility on the weekends.

If you follow healthy eating habits seven days a week, including weekends, it will be easier to maintain your weight successfully.

9. Stay hydrated

Drinking water is good for weight maintenance for several reasons. First, having a drink or two before a meal can help you feel fuller and control your calorie intake.

One study found that people who drank water before a meal consumed a 13% reduction in calories compared to participants who did not drink water. Additionally, drinking water has been shown to increase the calories you burn during the day slightly.

Drinking water regularly increases satiety and boosts metabolism, which are essential factors in weight maintenance.

10. Get enough sleep

Getting enough sleep has a significant impact on weight management. Lack of sleep is a major risk factor for weight gain in adults and can interfere with weight maintenance.

This is partly because sleep deprivation increases your appetite, which leads to higher levels of ghrelin, known as the hunger hormone. In addition, sleep-deprived people have lower levels of leptin, a hormone needed to regulate appetite.

In addition, people who sleep for a short period are simply tired and less motivated to exercise and choose healthy foods. If you're not getting enough sleep, find ways to change your sleeping habits. Getting at least 7 hours of sleep a night is optimal for weight management and overall health. Getting the right amount of sleep can help maintain weight by maintaining energy levels and keeping hormones in check.

11. Manage your stress levels

Stress management is an integral part of weight management. High-stress levels can contribute to weight gain by increasing cortisol levels, a hormone released in response to stress. Sustained increases in cortisol are associated with increased amounts of abdominal fat, increased appetite, and increased food intake.

Stress is also a common trigger for binge eating, especially when you're not hungry. Fortunately, there are many things you can do to relieve stress, including exercise, yoga, and meditation.

Controlling your stress levels is important for weight maintenance, as excessive stress can stimulate your appetite and increase your risk of weight gain.

12. Find a support system

Maintaining your weight goal can take time and effort. One strategy to overcome this is to find a support system that can work with you to take responsibility for a healthy lifestyle.

Some research suggests that having a friend to help you reach your goals can be helpful, especially if that person has a partner or spouse with similar healthy habits. One study looked at the health behaviors of more than 3,000 couples and found that when one partner adopts healthy habits, such as exercise, the other partner is more likely to follow suit.

Getting your partner or spouse involved in a healthy lifestyle increases your chances of maintaining your weight loss.

13. Monitor your food intake

People who record their food intake in a journal, online food tracker, or app are more likely to maintain their weight loss. Food trackers are helpful because they often provide accurate information about how many calories and nutrients you consume, making you more aware of your portion size. Additionally, various food trackers allow you to record your exercise so you can make sure you're eating the right amount to maintain your weight.

Here are some examples of websites and apps that count calories: Tracking what you eat each day lets you know how many calories and nutrients you're consuming, which can help you maintain your weight loss.

14. Eat enough vegetables

Several studies have linked increased vegetable consumption with improved weight management. First of all, vegetables are low in calories. You can eat large portions while getting plenty of nutrients without gaining weight. Vegetables are also rich in fiber, which increases satiety and automatically reduces the number of calories you consume during the day.

To reap these weight management benefits, eat one or two vegetables at every meal. Vegetables are high in fiber and low in calories. Both properties can help maintain weight.

15. Be consistent

Consistency is the key to maintaining your weight. Instead of going on a diet and returning to your old habits, it's better to stick with your new healthy diet and lifestyle forever.

Adopting a new lifestyle can initially seem daunting, but as you learn, making the right choices will become second nature. A healthy lifestyle will become easier, and weight maintenance will become easier.

It's easier to maintain your weight loss if you stick to your new healthy habits instead of going back to your old lifestyle.

16. Learn to eat wisely

Mindful eating is listening to your internal appetite signals and paying full attention to the eating process. This includes eating slowly and taking time to chew your food well so you can smell and taste it.

Eating this way makes you more likely to stop eating when you're full. Eating while distracted can make it challenging to recognize when you're full, leading to overeating.

Research shows that mindful eating can help maintain weight by targeting behaviors associated with weight gain, such as emotional eating.

Additionally, mindful eaters can maintain their weight without counting calories.

Mindful eating helps maintain weight because it helps you recognize fullness and prevents unhealthy behaviors that often lead to weight gain.

17. Make permanent changes in your lifestyle.

The reason most people fail to keep their weight off is that they follow unrealistic diets that don't work long-term.

They end up feeling deprived, which often causes them to gain more weight than they lost when they start eating normally again. Maintaining weight loss depends on permanently changing your lifestyle.

It looks different for everyone, but it means being consistent, not being too restrictive, and making the right choices as often as possible. Maintaining weight loss is easier if you make long-term lifestyle changes instead of following the unrealistic rules many weight loss diets focus on.

The Bottom Line

Diets can be restrictive, unrealistic and often lead to weight gain. But many simple changes to your habits can help you maintain long-term weight loss.

As you travel, you'll find that managing your weight involves more than what you eat. Exercise, sleep, and mental health also play an essential role.
Maintaining weight loss can be easier if you adopt a new lifestyle instead of continuing to try to lose weight with fad diets.

Sustainable lifestyle strategies.
Sustainable living refers to a way of life in which individuals or societies seek to reduce the use of the Earth's natural and personal resources.
For most of us, living an environmentally friendly life is something we strive to achieve daily. We can reduce the disposable items we use, recycle as much as possible, eat less meat and dairy, buy locally grown food in season, or walk instead of driving whenever possible.
At first glance, reducing carbon emissions may seem difficult. Especially when you see other people around you not doing their part. But when you break it down into small steps, you realize you have more power than you think To make sustainable living affordable,

12 ways to live a sustainable life
Every day, we make choices that affect our environment, climate, and other species. From the food we eat to the number of children we want, there are many things we can do to reduce

our carbon footprint by 'choosing wild' and leaving more room for animals and plants. Our actions matter.

- Think twice before you buy.
- Throw away plastic and recycle.
- Remove the plate from the plate.
- Makes vacations easier.
- Choose organic products.
- Avoid fast fashion and animal-based fabrics.
- Be careful with water.
- Drive less and be greener.
- Make your home green.
- Boycott products that pose a threat to wildlife.
- Fight for your right to choose when and if to start a family.
- Take action. Use your voice

1. Think twice before shopping.

Every product we buy has a carbon footprint, from the materials used to make it to the pollutants released during production to the packaging that ends up in landfills and incinerators. Even if you can recycle or compost a product at the end of its life, the damage has already been done. So before you buy something, ask yourself if you need it. If so, consider buying used rather than new and look for others that are made from low-impact materials and require less packaging and shipping costs.

2. Throw away the plastic and recycle.

Plastic will never go away. At least 14 million tonnes enter the ocean annually, equivalent to 80% of all marine debris. Every year, thousands of seabirds, sea turtles, seals, and other marine mammals die from ingesting plastic or drowning. You can reduce plastic waste by taking a few simple steps. Use reusable bags when shopping, throw away single-use water bottles, bags, and straws, and avoid products made or packaged in plastic as much as possible (for example, choose unpackaged products in supermarkets). Switch from single-use products to reusable ones. Every plastic-free product is a win for the planet.

3. Remove the plate from the plate.

Meat production is one of the most environmentally damaging industries in the world, responsible for massive amounts of water use, pollution, greenhouse gas emissions, and habitat destruction. So, eating more plant-based foods and less meat will also reduce your carbon footprint. Food is also the largest category of material dumped in municipal landfills. About 40 percent of the food we eat in the United States is wasted, along with all the land, water, and other natural resources used to produce it. Avoid food waste by shopping and planning wisely, and make sure you eat what you buy.

4. Rest comfortably during the holidays.

Holidays, birthdays, weddings, and other celebrations are often very extravagant. For example, Americans produce 23% more trash in December than any other month. But the problem is broader than excessive waste. With all the fossil fuels, trees, and other natural resources needed to produce gifts, decorations, disposable tableware, and wrapping paper, wildlife and their habitats overshadow our holidays. But you can redefine your vacation in a way that respects the land, water, and wildlife. Instead of celebrating your next holiday with plastic decorations, shiny gifts, and disposable food and drink containers, decorate with herbs, give homemade or thrifty gifts, and serve plant-based meals with reusable plates.

5. Choose organic.

From coffee to fruit to clothes, choosing organic products helps reduce the impact on nature and the planet. More than 2 billion pounds of pesticides are sold in the United States each year. Pesticides are widespread in fish and wildlife habitats, threatening the survival and recovery of hundreds of federally listed species. Pesticides also pollute the air, water, soil, and food. If you garden, avoid pesticides by growing organically at home. Creating wildlife in your yard by growing pollinator-friendly native plants and removing invasive species can help attract beneficial insects and ward off unwanted pests. Choosing green products helps keep harmful pesticides out of our land and water and protects farm workers, vulnerable communities, wildlife, and families.

6. Give up fast Fashion and animal prints.

Fast Fashion is a huge and fast-growing industry. Over the past 20 years, the number of new clothes created yearly has almost doubled, and global fashion consumption has increased by 400%. The fast fashion industry significantly contributes to the climate crisis and is responsible for 10% of global CO_2 emissions. Animal textiles such as wool cause water pollution, habitat loss from deforestation, and other damage to wildlife. Take care of your clothes, alter them whenever possible, and delay Fashion by shopping or exchanging if you need new clothes. If you must buy new clothes, go beyond greenwashing and buy clothes made from sustainable materials like organic cotton or Tencel from long-standing brands.

7. Be water-wise.

Water conservation has become critical as a growing population puts greater demands on the nation's water resources and faces unprecedented droughts. You can save water by reducing shower time, fixing toilet leaks, and choosing appliances that use less water and flow. Consider landscaping your garden with native, drought-adapted plants that require little water and maintenance over time and provide habitat and food for birds and bees. One of the biggest water hogs is cattle, so not eating meat and dairy also saves water.

8. Drive less and be greener.

Fuel vehicle emissions cause greenhouse gases, smoke, soot, and other harmful air pollution. But you can significantly reduce your carbon emissions by changing your driving habits. If possible, walk, cycle, drive, use public transport, or participate in walking or cycling. Consolidate your work to minimize travel. Participate or start a car-free day in your community. Ask local authorities to invest in electric parks and charging stations, and if you want to buy a new car, consider buying an electric car. It is also essential to keep your vehicle in good condition by regularly adjusting and inflating your tires. Gog increases fuel efficiency. A 20% underinflated tire can result in a 10% increase in your vehicle's fuel efficiency.

9. Make your home green.

Just as keeping your car in good condition improves gas mileage, keeping your home in good condition improves energy efficiency. Ensure your home is adequately insulated and has energy-efficient windows, use programmable thermostats for more efficient heating and cooling, and use CFLs for more efficient lighting. If your state allows you to choose your electricity supplier, use a company that generates at least half of its power from wind, solar, and other clean energy sources. Installing solar panels on your roof or installing a solar water heater will help the planet and save you money. Many states offer incentives to help you make your home greener or lower or lower your rent.

10. Boycott products that endanger wildlife.

In the United States, it is illegal to buy, sell, import, or sell products made from animals that are listed as endangered, but one's bottom line may be harmed even if the plant or animal in question is not listed. Some products also threaten endangered species in their habitats, from clearing old-growth forests to using water that coastal species need to survive. To avoid endangering wildlife, shop responsibly, look for products made from sustainable materials like bamboo, and eat at restaurants that don't serve endangered species like bluefin tuna.

11. Fight for the right to choose when and if to start a family.

The world's population is over 8 billion, and the demand for food, water, land, and fossil fuels is driving other species to extinction. Population growth and consumption underlie the most pressing environmental crises but are often ignored. By promoting reproductive health, rights and justice, and gender equality, we can improve the health of people and the planet as better education and access to family planning services reduce family size and the overall ecological footprint. Start the conversation by talking to your partner about family planning. Advocate for reproductive freedom in your community by advocating for free and easy access to comprehensive sexuality education, contraception, and abortion in schools.

12. Take action, use your voice.

One of the best things we can do for nature and our planet now and in the future is to become politically engaged at the community and national level. Vote for candidates with robust environmental platforms. Urge your representatives to adopt stronger policies to limit greenhouse gas emissions, combat climate change, protect wildlife and public lands, and support access to reproductive health. Talk with friends about the need to protect endangered species and fight overpopulation and overconsumption.

CONCLUSION

The journey to weight loss in a high-calorie world

Reflecting on Your Progress

Looking back at your accomplishments will show you how far you've come. Understanding how you've evolved (and how you can continue to evolve) can prepare you for future challenges.

Reflecting on your successes can be crucial to achieving your weight loss ambitions. Reflection can mean many things and varies from person to person, but setting new goals can be very effective. By exploring different reflection methods, you can decide which method is best for you. The reflection method

What went well?

Instead of focusing on what went wrong, celebrate what went right. Remember that change and progress do not happen overnight. Sometimes, positive change requires two steps forward and one step back. Celebrating these small events reinforces positive behavior, so celebrate them! Could you have found support in the right place? Or have you decided to eat healthy? Or have you lost a few inches even though you haven't lost any weight? These are all outstanding achievements that deserve to be celebrated.

What didn't work?

Did you spend two hours at the gym every morning before work, ate only 800 calories a day, and told yourself it took you a week to jump? You should limit yourself to one weight loss goal, such as working out on Monday, Wednesday, Friday, and Sunday, or getting more fiber into your diet by eating more fresh fruit and vegetables daily. Bad behavior happens over time. Therefore, it takes time to change unhealthy behaviors to healthy ones. Don't feel like you have to reevaluate everything in your life immediately. Instead, try to change one thing at a time. Don't decide what you "should" do or what others want from you. It should align with your values and goals. Think about it and prepare accordingly to change your lifestyle.

The power of journaling

Many people who set out to lose weight succeeded by keeping a journal and getting to know themselves better. Daily reflection on what works and what is not is half the battle. You may find that you crave salty foods when stressed, that eating out has a negative impact, or that stepping on the scale daily helps you feel more accountable. These so-called "key recommendations" help evaluate weight loss efforts and success in achieving future goals.

If you find it challenging to keep a diary, consider a food diary. Even if you're not consciously cutting calories or making healthy food choices, a food journal can help you track your eating habits. Many people keep a laptop or smartphone nearby and record everything they eat and drink throughout the day. Even if you write it down and throw it away, it keeps you accountable and is a very effective weight loss tool. It is also essential to regulate your emotions while eating.

The Importance Of Reflection

Purpose

Reflecting on your progress, especially when you reach your goals, gives you a sense of purpose, leading to happiness and productivity.

Improvement

Learning from unfulfilled goals means realizing where you are now and where you want to be. This can give you an idea of what you need to do to improve in the future.

Efficiency

Taking time out of your schedule to set goals can be very beneficial in the long run because it helps you plan your tasks and find the most efficient and effective ways to accomplish them.

Embrace a healthy and balanced life.

In today's busy world, it's easy to get confused and neglect your well-being. But to live a fulfilling life, you must take care of your physical, mental, and emotional health. A healthy lifestyle offers two benefits: not only does it improve our overall well-being, but it also allows us to live happier and more productive lives. We will explore some important aspects of a healthy lifestyle and learn how to incorporate them into everyday life.

Maintain a balanced and nutritious diet.

It is necessary to form a healthy lifestyle. What we feed our bodies has a direct impact on our energy levels, immune system, and overall vitality. By choosing whole foods such as fruits, vegetables, whole grains, and lean proteins, we can ensure that we get a variety of essential nutrients. In addition, it is important to stay hydrated by drinking enough water for our body to function optimally.

Regular physical activity.

Regular exercise can provide several important benefits. Not only does it help maintain weight, but it also improves cardiovascular health, strengthens muscles, and improves mood. Finding an activity you enjoy, such as running, swimming, dancing, or yoga, can make it easier to incorporate exercise into your daily routine. Furthermore, even small changes, such as taking the stairs instead of the elevator or a brisk walk during lunch, can have a positive impact on our health and overall well-being.

Adequate rest and sleep.

It is important for our health. Unfortunately, in today's fast-paced modern world, good sleep takes second place in our lives. However, sleep and rest are the building blocks of a healthy mind and body. Because while we sleep, our bodies repair and rejuvenate, and our minds process information and consolidate memories. That's why we need to make good sleep a priority to give our bodies the energy that leads to increased productivity, improved cognitive function, and a stronger immune system.

It is also important to understand that maintaining a healthy lifestyle is not limited to the physical areas of our body and that taking care of our mental and emotional well-being is just as important. Managing your stress levels plays an important role in your overall health. Especially in today's stressful world, we must engage in stress-reducing activities such as meditation, deep breathing, and mindfulness exercises. In addition, we can maintain good relationships and seek support from loved ones, which gives us a sense of belonging and contributes to our emotional well-being.

Living a healthy lifestyle is a journey, not a destination. Bringing about positive change requires persistence, dedication, and will. By developing healthy habits and incorporating them into our daily lives, we can reap the long-term benefits of better physical health, mental well-being, and greater satisfaction. Ultimately, a healthy lifestyle begins with self-awareness and a willingness to make positive changes. It's about valuing ourselves enough to prioritize our happiness and making conscious choices that support our overall health. So, let's all take the first step today and begin the journey to a healthier, happier, and more fulfilling life. We must never forget. A healthy lifestyle is not a luxury. It's an investment in ourselves and our future well-being!